THE UNSEEN
TERRORIST

THE UNSEEN TERRORIST

OCHE OTORKPA

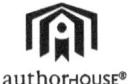

authorHOUSE®

AuthorHouse™ UK Ltd.
1663 Liberty Drive
Bloomington, IN 47403 USA
www.authorhouse.co.uk
Phone: 0800.197.4150

Published by AuthorHouse 12/09/2013

ISBN: 978-1-4918-8738-7 (sc)
ISBN: 978-1-4918-8740-0 (hc)
ISBN: 978-1-4918-8739-4 (e)

DEDICATION

To the individuals and families whose stories
I have shared in this book.

CONTENTS

ACKNOWLEDGEMENTS

My deepest appreciation goes to all those whose stories I have shared in this book and the families that have shared their pains with the hope that our society will be a better place by the sacrifices they have made.

To all those who have taken time to painstakingly go through this work, I will forever remain indebted.

Special thanks to my family for their love, patience and encouragement.

This book is a collection of true life stories to which fictional names and characters have been assigned to protect the identity of the victims and individuals.

INTRODUCTION

By the time you go through the first five lines of this book, one person would have been infected with the HIV virus. With millions of death and new infections every year, the world is under siege by a sea of animalcules.

From June 5th 1981 when the first case of HIV/AIDS was reported, the prevalence rate of the disease has continued to undulate in an orographic manner in different regions of the world.

Daily, thousands of young people become infected worldwide. A disturbing aspect of the UN's yearly report on HIV/AIDS is the fact that women and young people continue to account for a large percentage of new infections. Despite this high prevalence rate, 9 out of 10 infected persons globally do not know they carry the virus. In the United States for example, women account for 1in 5 new HIV diagnoses and deaths caused by AIDS with a vast majority contracting the virus through heterosexual sex. With infection rates in Australia at a twenty year high and over thirty percent increase in the number of people infected with drug resistant strains of the virus in Europe, there is virtually no continent unaffected by the pandemic.

The Russian federation with one of the highest rates of HIV infections after sub Saharan Africa is battling with a new and more virulent strain of the virus, while the Chinese emerged from an era of denialism and contaminated blood scandals to confront an epidemic that is threatening to incapacitate its young and inexpensive labour force which it heavily relies upon to drive its rapidly growing economy.

In Southern Africa, entire communities have been wiped out of the map, while grandmothers are left with the burden of caring for orphans whose parents have been consumed by the rampaging virus. The story is not different in East Africa, where the virus has redrawn the map of several communities. For Bernadette Nakayima, a Ugandan grandmother who lost all of her 11 children to AIDS and now cares for 35 grand children no disease can be more cruel.

In sub-Saharan Africa, where AIDS is responsible for 1 out of every 5 deaths, the Gross Domestic Product (GDP) of most countries continue to slide, not just because of bad governance, mismanagement and corruption but also to a large extent due to the impact of HIV/AIDS on young people trained in various field of human endeavour but rendered useless to their countries and communities by a virus that continues to terrorise humanity.

The issue surrounding HIV/AIDS are deeply embedded in socio-cultural beliefs and practices many of them intimate, personal and private. From Ethiopia in the horn of Africa to the Cape of Good Hope in South Africa, from London in the West to Beijing the heart of Asia, a terrorist is on the loose, redefining the course of human existence.

This book is a collection of short stories, my experiences and interaction with communities in the struggle to tame the virus, which is meant to elicit a cross sectional discuss on the strategies we employ in the fight against a common enemy.

HIV AIDS is a disease with stigma. And we have learned with experience not just with HIVAIDS but with other diseases, countries for many reasons are sometimes hesitant to admit they have a problem.

—**Magareth Chan**

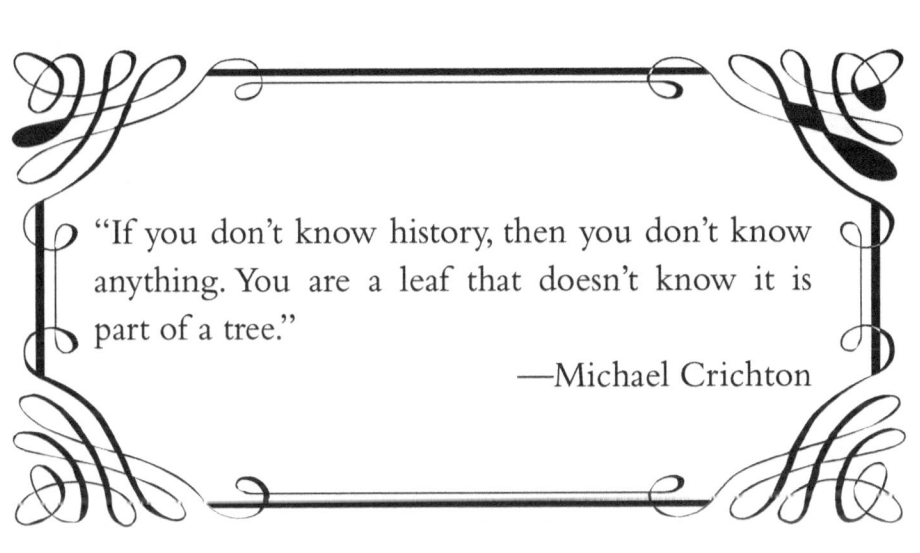

"If you don't know history, then you don't know anything. You are a leaf that doesn't know it is part of a tree."

—Michael Crichton

HIV: HIS-STORY

Till date, the origin of HIV/AIDS continues to be shrouded in deep controversy with two schools of thought locked in a war for supremacy, with the battle showing no signs of abating. To fully understand the history of HIV/AIDS, the summary of both schools of thought is presented below.

SCHOOL OF MUTATION

This school of thought tries to promote the idea that the virus was a product of mutation (transformation) of the Simian Immuno Deficiency Virus SIV 1 and 2 found in African monkeys, especially the African green monkey. This virus has characteristics similar to that of the human immunodeficiency virus HIV 1 and 2, the causative agent of AIDS

SCHOOL OF NAOMI

This second school of thought promotes the belief in the plot to systematically control the population of blacks with a special virus programme commissioned by the United States Government in the last century code named M.K-NAOMI decoded as follows

M = Robert Manaker

K = Paul Kotin

Names of the 2 researchers, who authored the virus.

N = Negroes (Black's)

A = Are

O = Only

M = Momentary

I = Individuals

Proponents of this idea believe this programme led to the production of the lethal virus HIV, proliferated as complement of the small pox vaccine for Africa and "experimental" Hepatitis B vaccine for Manhattan as a result of which many blacks and homosexuals became victims.

Whichever side of the divide you belong is not as important as your resolve for a collective action against a disease that continues to defy human wisdom.

However, the efforts of some individuals in trying to deny the existence of the virus despite overwhelming scientific and physical evidence to the contrary is perhaps one of the greatest challenge facing care givers and advocacy groups around the globe.

This is because the action of these denialists and dissident HIV scientists created the perfect atmosphere that brought about the policy summersault in South Africa which led to the death of over three hundred thousand (3000,000) people according to a Harvard research in 2008. This is a part of history most scientists, activists, and care givers would rather not talk about.

Quote: *"The greatest grand challenge for any scientist is discovering how to prevent the spread of HIV and finding the cure or an effective vaccine for AIDS"*

—Philip Emeagwali

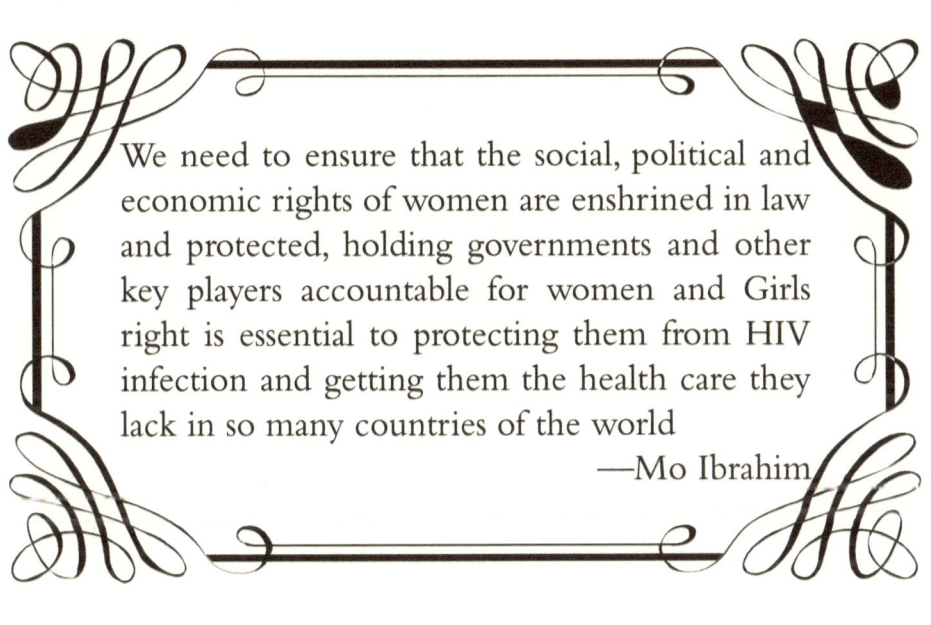

We need to ensure that the social, political and economic rights of women are enshrined in law and protected, holding governments and other key players accountable for women and Girls right is essential to protecting them from HIV infection and getting them the health care they lack in so many countries of the world

—Mo Ibrahim

DRIVING WOMEN TO EXTINCTION

Hajia Maimuna is a caring mother, a good wife, an excellent entrepreneur, and a Gold merchant. On the 5th of August few years ago while travelling to Abuja Nigeria's capital city, the vehicle she was travelling in was Blocked by dare devil armed robbers disguised as military men who stripped her of all she had; money, gold and precious ornaments. This hard working lady was bruised, battered, raped and dumped by the road side to die.

When Pricillia, a newly recruited banker boarded a tricycle at the close of work, little did she know that the events that would unfold over the next four hours would change her life forever. It was about 7:35 pm when she left the bank after a long day of debiting and crediting accounts, hopping into the next available tricycle. Mid way into the ride, other passengers alighted at different bus stops leaving Pricillia and the driver. The decisive moment came when the driver on the excuse of avoiding the usually heavy traffic along Douglas road in Owerri, South East Nigeria, took a detour and ended in an obscure location where he raped Pricilla at gun point, took her mobile phones and disappeared into thick darkness.

Few weeks later Pricillia was at the Federal Medical Center Owerri to complain of the side effects of the drugs she was given as Post Exposure Prophylaxis (PEP) for HIV. That was when the unimaginable happened. As Pricillia walked away from the pharmacy, she saw a man having a striking resemblance with the fellow who raped her; he was dropping some relatives who had come to see a patient at the hospital. As she moved closer, she could not believe her eyes; she was standing face to face with the man who took her most priced asset in a cruel and dehumanizing manner. Convinced that she had the right man, she grabbed his shirt and alerted passersby who gathered within minutes.

As Pricillia narrated her ordeal the man denied the accusation insisting he had nothing to do with her predicament and should be excused, that was when she made a statement that stunned the crowed.

She said, "the man who raped me has a big scar on his thigh, so if you show these people your thighs and there is no scar I will apologize and let you go"

At this point, a larger crowd had gathered but the driver was not willing to pull down his trousers in full glare of the public, until a policeman showed up. When he pulled down his trousers, a loud noise erupted as the crowd descended on the man beating him up mercilessly.

The hidden scar had exposed him as the man who raped an innocent lady on her way back from the office.

Many disciplined and hard working women have innocently fallen prey to the activities of these hoodlums whose appetite for hard drugs and rape of innocent girls and women have continued to defy solutions.

Raped at age nine by a relative and pregnant at 14 Oprah Winfrey, like many others have experienced the wickedness and brutality of our society. Sadly, it's an environment where blood lines no longer hold.

Increasingly, the girl child is becoming an endangered specie as pedophiles' continue to roam free in our societies terrorizing the lives of our children and stripping them of all the joy and excitement that comes with childhood.

From New Delhi to New York, from Durban to Rio; women and girls are been hunted down by rapists, abused by pedophiles and emotionally decapitated by a society that is becoming increasingly hostile to the womenfolk.

Quote: "*we need a deep social revolution that will give more power to women, and transform relations between women and men at all levels of society. It is only when 'women can speak up, and have a full say in decisions affecting their lives, that they will be able to truly protect themselves and their children-against HIV*"

—**Kofi Annan**

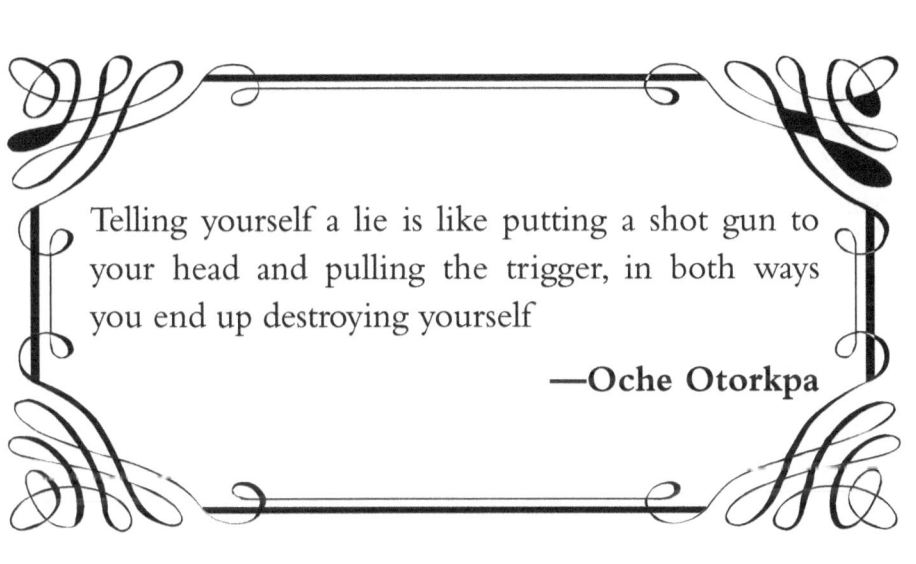

Telling yourself a lie is like putting a shot gun to your head and pulling the trigger, in both ways you end up destroying yourself

—Oche Otorkpa

PLAYBOY PATHWAY

Junior was thirteen years old, when he had his first sexual intercourse with a neighbour's daughter Mary, who was 4 years older. From then onwards Junior never looked back as he jumped from one girl to another.

Despite becoming sexually active as a Junior Secondary School II student, Junior's academic brilliance was a source of great joy to his parents, his performance at Senior Secondary school Certificate Examination (SSCE), was the best in recent times and as the only child of his parents, he received every encouragement and got admitted into the Law Faculty of the Obafemi Awolowo University Ile-Ife, South-west Nigeria. Even as a freshman he continued to maintain his status as Play boy 001, the ultimate chick magnet and the boy every freshman and sophomore wanted to be like. It was a strong belief by most guys on campus that Junior had a "God-given" charm which made him irresistible to any girl regardless of her class.

He graduated from University with good grades and proceeded to the Nigerian Law School. He did very well at law school and then proceeded for the mandatory one year National Youth Service—all these while junior's lucky streak with the ladies continued.

However, two weeks to his passing out Parade and subsequent move to England for post graduate studies, nemesis came knocking at the door. Junior became ill and was hospitalized for seven days. He could neither eat nor drink and everyone was terrified at the alarming rate at which he lost weight.

At the hospital, the doctor asked to see Junior's relatives, by this time Junior's parents had arrived having been informed earlier of his worsening health condition by the corper's liaison officer (CLO).

After spending some time at his bed side, His parents were ushered into the doctor's office. In the office, the doctor's major problem was not Junior but his mother who was crying profusely not believing what her eyes had seen, and lamenting the fate that could befall her only child, yet the doctor was about to reveal the mystery behind her son's ill health.

While similar events have become a characteristic of our generation no one seems to be noticing. Universities and College hostels have been transformed to be mini brothels while "roaming" after school is fast becoming a tradition among secondary or high school students.

For peanuts young men are willing to sacrifice their lives on the altar of pleasure, taking on women old enough to be their mothers.

The "Play Boy" syndrome has come to be accepted in most communities as a way of life. While the boys see it as the height of their romantic illusion, the girls are happy to jump at any offer from the ladies man not minding the consequences.

The fact that a play boy and his lieutenants could become victims of HIV/AIDS and STIs, be assaulted by an estranged lover or lose future ability to differentiate between true love and infatuation seem not to be a source of worry, neither does unwanted pregnancy, child birth or abortion which could stop education and eventually lead to a low self esteem appear to deter many.

As the world confronts the challenges of globalisation, the entertainment Industry and a web saturated with explicit sexual content, is increasingly making it difficult for young people to make informed decisions about sex, the media simply encourage young lads to make potentially dangerous decisions completely denying them of the right to know the consequences of those actions. As T.D Jakes rightly puts it "life will always require us to take risks but we must discern which risk is worth taking and which will short circuit our long term goals for short term pleasure".

It is important to note that while the expression of one's sexuality is a normal component of living, control over this natural phenomenon is however an individual decision. This is where Sex Education comes in. But are parents ready to take on the taboo subject?

Quote:

"Players" are liable to die young"

—*Oche Otorkpa*

PLAYBOY PATHWAY

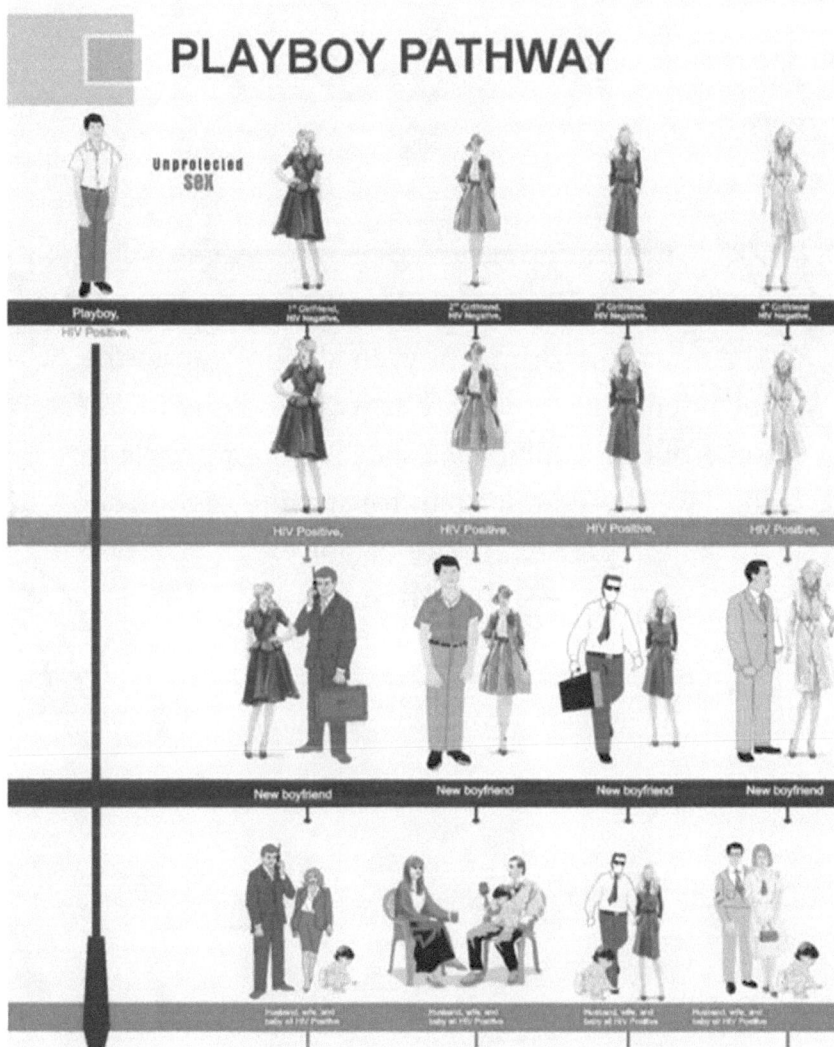

Unprotected sex

Playboy, HIV Positive,

1st Girlfriend, HIV Negative,

2nd Girlfriend, HIV Negative,

3rd Girlfriend, HIV Negative,

4th Girlfriend, HIV Negative,

HIV Positive,

HIV Positive,

HIV Positive,

HIV Positive,

New boyfriend

New boyfriend

New boyfriend

New boyfriend

Husband, wife, and baby all HIV Positive

Husband, wife, and baby all HIV Positive

Husband, wife, and baby all HIV Positive

Husband, wife, and baby all HIV Positive

Death

: "Anyway, no drug, not even alcohol, causes the fundamental ills of society. If we're looking for the source of our troubles, we shouldn't test people for drugs, we should test them for stupidity, ignorance, greed and love of power".

—P.J. O'Rourke

CLOUD NINE

During the Navratri Festival in Baroda Gujarat State, West of India. I was amazed by warmth of the people and display of a high sense of decorum and responsibility by the youths especially the young men.

The festival was completely devoid of the irresponsible display of masculinity despite the large turnout of young women. This is in sharp contrast to what happens during festivals in Africa and many other parts of the world where it is increasingly becoming popular to sell Alcohol and hard drugs in pre-packed syringes and casings to young people, who end up destroying themselves and completely defeating the essence of such festivals.

As a student at Sultan Bello Secondary school, Sokoto, during the early 90s, I have experienced firsthand how easy it is for a ten year old to obtain marijuana for next to nothing, this trend seems to have been taken to a new dimension with the abuse of pharmaceutical products especially prescription medicines in schools and communities, increasing the number of mentally and emotionally challenged men and women on our streets and diverting young people from classrooms and lecture halls to prisons and drug rehabilitation centers.

Never in the history of mankind was the use of hard drugs so widespread, that despite the increasing risk of HIV, Endocarditis and drug induced psychosis, the number of drug addicts in developed and developing countries have continued to swell.

HIV infection associated with injection drug use is becoming a public health crisis largely due to the increased use of heroin and cocaine among young people.

According to the World Health Organization (WHO), about 16 million people inject drugs globally and 3 million of them are living with HIV. On average, one out of every ten new HIV infections is caused by injecting drug use. In parts of Eastern Europe and Central Asia over 80 percent of all HIV infections is related to drug use.

Drug cartels have taken the driver's seat, training our young men and women on how best to self destruct, while the larger community watches on helplessly as these bands of renegades lead our people towards the path of self annihilation.

In their quest to hit cloud Nine, our young men and women in their prime are gradually finding themselves on ground Zero, emotionally battered, academically bankrupt and medically paralyzed.

Quote

"I think if you were Satan and you were seating around trying to think up something that would just bring the human race to its knees what you would probably come up with is narcotics."

—**Cormac McCarthy**

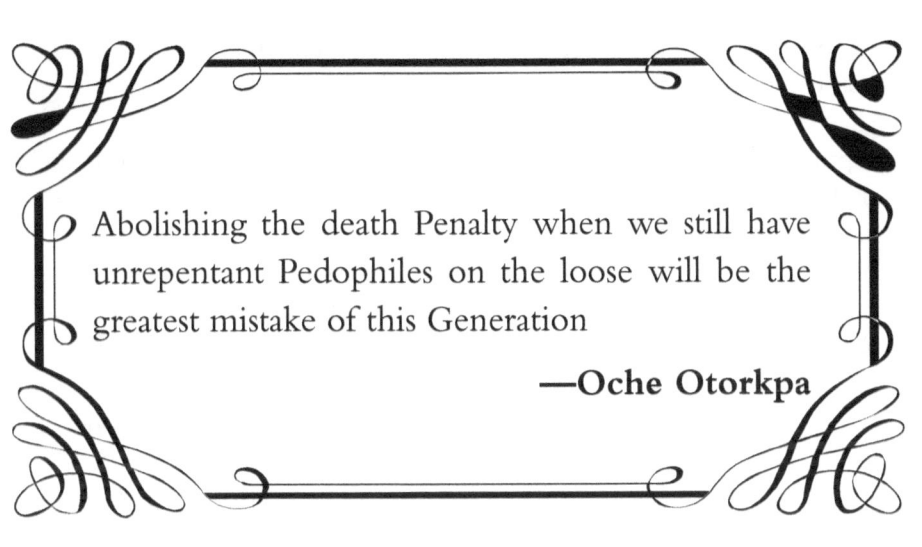

Abolishing the death Penalty when we still have unrepentant Pedophiles on the loose will be the greatest mistake of this Generation

—Oche Otorkpa

HUNTING FOR PEDOPHILES

Mrs. Winifred left for the shopping mall, beaming with smiles, the mall had just taken delivery of new stocks, and among them was an Italian leather handbag she had coveted for a long time. She had been saving for long in the hope of buying the high quality handbag to match her new status as an assistant manager at a drug manufacturing firm.

Upon receiving the news of the new arrivals from a friend, she dashed to the nearest automated teller machine to make withdrawals and hastily boarded a taxi heading for the mall. Her joy knew no bounds as she picked the bag, strolling majestically towards the counter where she paid for the bag and joyfully headed home to share the news with her husband who was on a weeklong sick leave.

As she opened the door, the sight of her husband sexually abusing their one year old daughter was more than she could take, she suddenly collapsed on the floor smashing her head on a glass stool as she made her way down.

Rushed to a nearby hospital, she was resuscitated but waking up to the reality that she has been married to a beast for ten years.

Over the years, as I recall these episodes, my heart bleeds. As a guide who works closely with children and young people it grieves my heart to see the pain our society continues to inflict on the vulnerable and defenseless.

The media is flooded with horrific stories and images of the continuous violation and molestation of our children from fathers who destroy their babies to randy Priests who defile the temple, our environment is completely ensnared.

The media itself is not left out of this onslaught against our children. The increased sexualization and eroticalization of our kids by the media has been identified as a major contributing factor to the way girls view sexuality. The promotion of appearance and physical attractiveness as key values by the media has also been implicated as one of the leading cause of eating disorders, depression and low self esteem among young people.

To the few who survived these brutal onslaught, the scars as well as the emotional and psychological trauma remain and continue to torment them destroying their self esteem, and changing their view and perception of society as they journey through life. It is therefore imperative to canvass for legislations that are stiff enough to serve as a nightmare for pedophiles and would be child molesters.

According to the FBI, 61 percent of rape victims are under 18 and 29 percent are younger than 11 yet only 1 out of every 10 child sexual abuse is reported to law enforcement agents.

The lack of stringent laws and the inefficient prosecution of perpetrators have made it increasingly difficult for victims and their families to get the justice they deserve.

In the absence of a global tracking system to effectively track pedophiles and checkmate their activities, the door will continue to remain open to these group of people who sneak into Facebook, connect with us on Twitter and show the world how they violated and infected our children on YouTube.

Quote

"To ask people not only to believe in the abuse but also to take on board all the details of what I'm revealing is a big step, and it has taken me many years to make the decision to tell my story, but it has to be done. This type of abuse is ongoing, as is the culture of disbelief to make people dismiss anyone who talks about it. This needs to be challenged. The things I'm telling you in this book have been kept close to me all my life; I have always

known that talking of them, telling my full story, would make some people incredulous—but it's true. It's all true.

Whatever the set dressing, they were rapists and abusers—just plain and simple/The trappings that surrounded the abuse was just a way of creating something that would allow them to do what they wanted to, but which would also allow for confusion on our parts, and devotion on the parts of the 'followers'. I think this is what many people find so hard when they are asked to believe in this sort of abuse. It all seems so fantastical, so it's easy to dismiss. I'm not asking you to believe in any of that. I'm not asking you to believe in Satan, I'm not even asking you to believe in God. I'm just asking you to accept that there are some people who will go to extraordinary lengths to cover up the facts that they are abusing children."

—**Laurie Matthew**

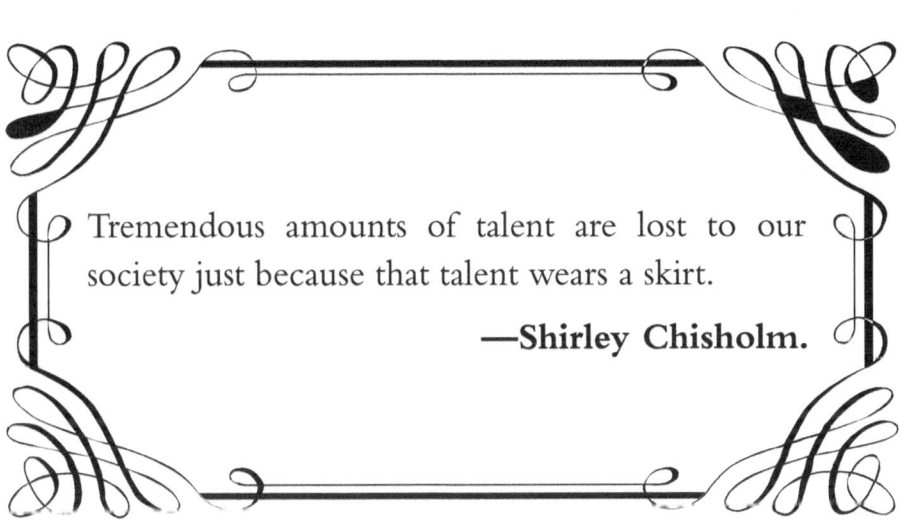

Tremendous amounts of talent are lost to our society just because that talent wears a skirt.

—**Shirley Chisholm.**

SKIRTPHILIA

Muyiwa a civil servant has just been transferred from Lagos, South West Nigeria to Abuja the nation's capital city, a womanizer to the core; Muyiwa did not spare anything in skirt.

As a routine, he comes home with different ladies who cook and keep his bed warm in the absence of his wife who was several miles away in Lagos.

However, the event of 18th July same year marked a turning point in the life of this father of three.

On arrival from work that hot Monday afternoon, he discovered that the young lady who had kept his bed warm for two weeks was nowhere to be found. To compound issues a note was left on the table which reads *"AIDS IS REAL"*. After 3 sleepless nights and a query from his boss, Muyiwa decided to go for a HIV test and the result came out negative, but that was not all, He was expected back at the clinic in six months time for a repeat test.

During the wait, Muyiwa's behaviour became very irrational. When the second test was carried out six months later, the story was a different one. Muyiwa was now HIV positive, and he lost his job 2 weeks later.

While some of us are so blind we could "toast" a Scottish man in kilt, others blinded by their desire for skirts continue to infect their loved ones with the virus they picked up from the usual all night "business meetings". It's sad that a lot of men go into marriages without the intention of keeping those vows. As the head of the home it is the duty of the man to protect his family from any form of aggression be it physical or biological.

Globally, millions of married men and women engage the services of sex workers each year. Despite growing health concerns about the increased risk of STDs and HIV AIDS this trade continues to blossom, leading to the premature termination of several lives and the dissolution of several marriages. But why should we continue to eat sour grapes?

Quote:

"HIV is free, why pay for it"

—**Oche Otorkpa**

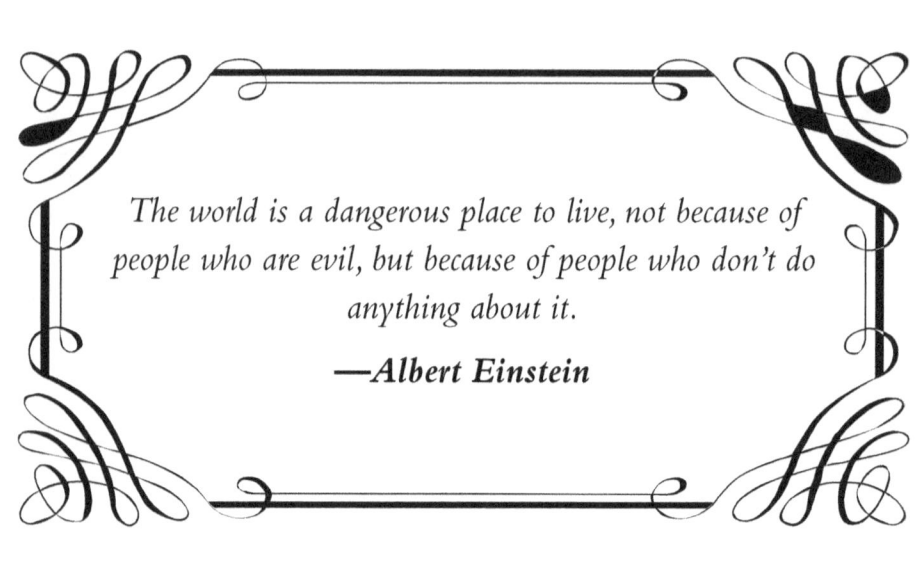

The world is a dangerous place to live, not because of people who are evil, but because of people who don't do anything about it.

—Albert Einstein

THE EVIL CLAN

When lab results showed that Emeka was infected with the HIV virus, members of his immediate family strategized on how to take care of him. After series of meetings and consultations, they came to the "brilliant" conclusion that keeping the information secret was in the best interest of the clan. Secondly, they decided to find a suitable bride, who would take care of him when he becomes weaker and unable to do most things by himself, since the demand of their business will not permit them to do so.

Ezinne, the daughter of Mazi Ikenna, a poor farmer from the neighboring village of Ogbeotu was picked for the assignment. Unknown to Ezinne and members of her family, they were being lured into a scheme that would have lethal consequences.

Several months after the wedding, Emeka began to show physical signs of the disease and was admitted for few weeks at a local hospital. Ezinne who was already seven months pregnant by this time was always at his bed side taking care of his needs to the "delight" of his family members.

As his health deteriorated, Ezinne had to virtually do everything for her husband as he could neither speak nor stand without support. He eventually died on the 5th of September exactly 18 months after the wedding and was hastily buried by his family.

Two months later when Ezinne his wife put to bed, none of her husband's relatives showed up to rejoice with her on the birth of her daughter. As the widow settled down to raise her daughter, her husband's relatives sold the only house her husband left and shared the money among themselves leaving her and her little child with no shelter.

Forced to relocate to her father's house, Ezinne, whose health was already failing struggled to take care of her daughter who was also HIV positive. With frequent hospital visits and mounting medical bills draining the family's finances, her father started asking questions.

He was later to discover the grand set up that transformed Ezinne his daughter into a guinea pig for Emeka's family. However, being financially handicapped to seek judicial redress, he sold as much farm produce as he could to pay the medical bills of his daughter's and her child.

As Ezinne narrated her ordeal to me on her hospital bed, tears rolled down her eyes as she clutched a picture of her dead child to her chest.

As I left her ward that evening, I wondered how many innocent young brides would have to die before the authorities take action.

Quote:

When I despair, I remember that all through history the way of truth and love have always won. There have been tyrants and murderers, and for a time, they can seem invincible but in the end they will always fall. Think of it—always

—**Mahatma Gandhi**

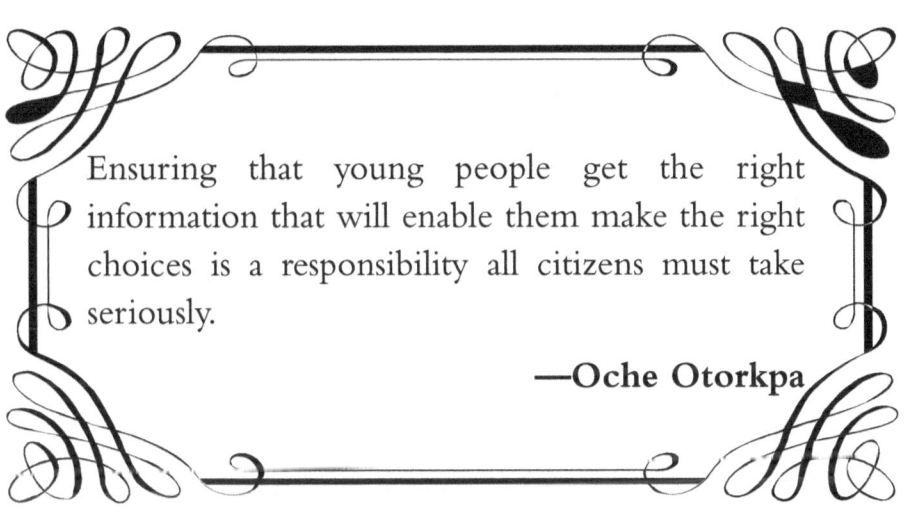

Ensuring that young people get the right information that will enable them make the right choices is a responsibility all citizens must take seriously.

—**Oche Otorkpa**

DRIVERS LOUNGE

The following conversation took place between a passer-by and a young girl about 14 years old, who was crying near a motor park.

Passer-by: why are you crying?

Young girl: *na my boflend* (it is my boyfriend).

Passer-by: Ah! You mean your boyfriend.

Young girl: *Ehn* (yes) still sobbing.

Passer-by: What happened?

Young girl: *I tell am say I don cally belle `ekon say make I go give my mama* (I told him I was pregnant and he said I should go and give the pregnancy to my mother)

This teenage girl was impregnated by a truck driver at a park where she hawks packaged water and soft drinks for someone she calls *antee* (aunty) a relative who brought her from the village several years ago. Like many other terrorists, these drivers simply disappear from the park and reappear at another park with a clean slate leaving their victims mostly children to fend for themselves. The denial of the pregnancy by the driver raises some difficult questions;

> ➢ What will happen to this girl when she returns home?

> ➢ If sent away, where will she seek refuge?

> ➢ What will happen to the unborn child?

> ➢ What if she had contracted the virus?

Daily young girls of school age find themselves in situations that render them vulnerable to all kinds of exploitation. In the United States for example,

➢ 4 in 10 girls become pregnant before the age of 20.

➢ Only 4 out of 10 teen mothers finish high school.

➢ Nearly 80% of fathers do not marry the teen mothers of their children.

➢ Only 30% of teenage mothers who marry after their child is born remain in those marriages.

The picture is not different in other parts of the world, especially Latin America and Africa where teenage pregnancy is booming, diverting children from schools to antenatal clinics and baby factories. The prevalence of wars, civil strife, harmful traditional practices, and extreme poverty only points to one fact, the world is saturated with children most of whom will be deprived of the right of been nurtured by the side of their own fathers.

Quote:

"The sexual abuse and exploitation of children is one of the most vicious crimes conceivable, a violation of mankind's most basic duty to protect the innocent"

—*James T. Walsh*

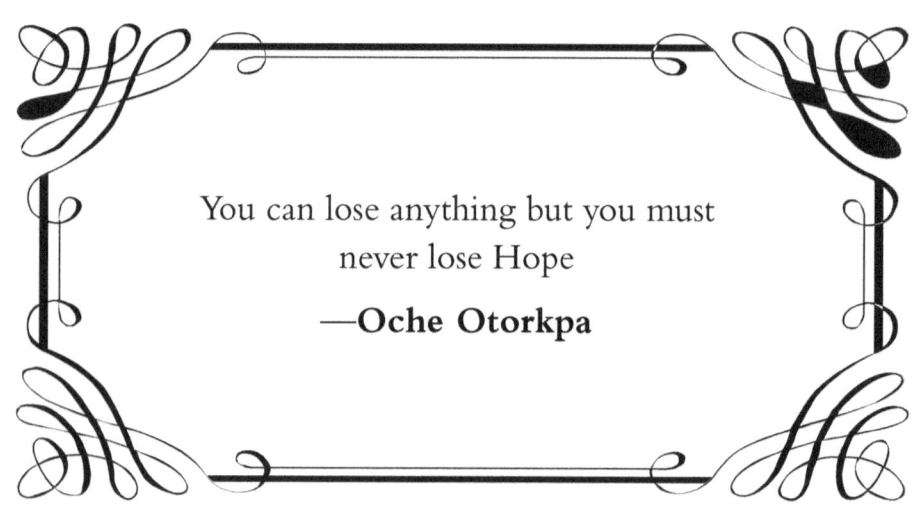

You can lose anything but you must
never lose Hope

—Oche Otorkpa

WHEN NOT TO SHARE GRACE

Efe was eighteen years old when I met her for the first time while traveling on a bus to Lokoja North Central, Nigeria. She had bright eyes and was full of life but deep beneath the light skin and radiant face was a story of pain, bitterness and love.

On a visit to her house few years ago, I noticed an unusual tattoo on her wrist that got me curious and I asked *"wetin de your hand sef"* (what's that on your hand?) And she replied

"It's a long story and I don't want to talk about it anymore" as she opened the fridge at the corner of the living room.

As I settled down into the soft leather sofa with a glass of orange juice in front of me, Efe emerged from the kitchen, walked straight to me and asked why I was interested on the scorpion tattooed to her wrist and I simply told her I was scared of people with tattoos, she smiled and said "finish your drink and I will tell you everything".

"About ten years ago after the death of my father, my mother took me to Aunty Evelyn her cousin in Gusau, Zamfara state, North West Nigeria. I was about 12 years old. *Madam* as Aunty Evelyn was called treated me very well; she changed my cloths and enrolled me at a private school few meters away from her house. My joy knew no bounds as I quickly settled into my new environment.

Aunty had a very big restaurant where she sold food and alcohol. The business was booming, and the men who came to eat or drink at our place will often give us money.

Our restaurant was well organized, everyone of the over 20 girls knew what was expected of each of them, apart from the occasional girl quarrel everything was perfect, until the State Government introduce the Sharia legal system (Islamic law).

The system brought about a sudden shut down of all premises where alcohol was sold. The alcohol business was the livewire of our restaurant; its ban completely crippled our business. For several months, we watched as our once bustling restaurant and bar became a warehouse for chairs and tables while Aunty became increasingly hostile as her business fortune dwindled.

One Friday afternoon, Aunty summoned a meeting and informed everyone that she was leaving town and closing the restaurant for good, this did not come to me as a surprise as I had previously heard her discussing with a lady over the phone about her plans to relocate.

Forty eight hours later, Aunty instructed the girls to pack, selecting twelve of them to make the trip with us while others returned to their families.

Fourteen of us including aunty left the city that night aboard a Mercedes 911 truck which carried all our belongings and headed for the garden city of Port Harcourt South of Nigeria. After a long tortuous journey, we finally arrived a city bustling with life and littered with expatriate oil workers who had lots of petro dollars, Aunty had secured the perfect environment to re-launch her businesses I said to myself.

Two days after our arrival, our sleep was disrupted by a loud bang on our door, it was about 2 am in the morning and we were terrified, but our fear soon gave way as we heard the voice of Aunty Evelyn asking all the girls to move to her room.

As we stepped into her room, the sight of a middle aged woman in white cloth seating over a big black pot sent further shock waves down our spines. On noticing the fear on our faces, Aunty quickly calmed our nerves by introducing us one after the other to the lady who immediately proceeded with the ceremony.

One after the other, the girls took turn to swear the oath of allegiance to Aunty and Ohe, the goddess of the night. the consequence of violating the oath was slow and painful death.

When I woke up that morning, I realized my legs were swollen; my body was probably reacting to the concoction we had taken the previous night before the scorpion was tattooed to our wrists. Nevertheless, I soon joined the girls to entertain the white men who had visited our lodge to welcome us to the city.

The white men had lots of dollars, and always lavished gifts and money on any girl who goes the extra mile to satisfy their lust. As the years rolled by we slept with men of all shades and characters, remitting eighty percent of our proceeds to Aunty. The oil workers ensured we lacked nothing. Life was good or so we thought, until Mene died.

Mene was my best friend, she had been sick for two days and suddenly died on the third, we had all expected her to pull through, but she never did.

Aunty did not allow us mourn as Mene was quickly buried at a nearby bush and life continued as if nothing had happened.

It was Mene's death that pushed me into deep reflections; I became lonely and depressed as I pondered over what had happened. Mene had disagreed with Aunty a few days earlier over the fees we remit. Could aunty have murdered my best friend? As wild thoughts ran through my mind, I started planning my escape, and with every passing day I dreamt of the day when I will be free from the clutches of the Ohe deity.

As I made my plans, I realized I would need some help if my dream was to become a reality, so I shared my plot with a fellow roommate Ada, who made me believe she also wanted out only to reveal my plans to Aunty.

I was in the market, buying food stuffs for the lodge when I received a text message from Ovie Aunty Evelyn's former boyfriend that Ada had revealed my escape plans to Aunty. Straight up I knew I had to activate my plan ahead of schedule, going back to the lodge was not an option.

Armed with the money to buy food stuffs, I headed for the motor park. That day was the last time I saw Aunty. I boarded a vehicle heading to Abuja Nigeria's capital city. The journey was very smooth and we arrived Abuja some few minutes before midnight. As other passengers disappeared into the darkness I searched for a spot where I could lay my head till the next day.

As the cockcrow signaled the birth of a new day, I moved round the park in a bid to get familiar with my new environment which was already bustling with life as tea sellers and restaurants light up their fire place to prepare for the day's business.

As I moved round I stumbled on an advert at a restaurant within the park which read, Sales girl wanted; apply in person. That was my perfect opportunity, I applied immediately and started work same day.

As night falls and the once bustling motor park goes quiet I and other workers spread our mats on the floor of the restaurant which also served as our bedroom at night. My new *madam* was kind to me and her business prospered under my watch.

I never knew my HIV status until Victor proposed to me and we had to do some laboratory test as a pre requisite for the announcement of our wedding banns at our local church.

Despite the fact that the result came back positive, Victor still went ahead and married me and today I have a son for him who is HIV negative, we received extensive counseling at the clinic when I tested positive and continued to receive support even after the birth of my son. Victor, my husband knew all I had gone through and was willing to support me all through.

Today, I have my own restaurant, a bundle of joy as a son and a wonderful, caring and understanding husband. Heaven has been kind to me, Oche"

As I left her apartment that evening, I recall the words of my mathematics teacher, Mr Rene, who said "every problem has a solution"

Quote

"Being deeply loved by someone gives you strength, while loving someone deeply gives you courage."

—**Lao Tzu**

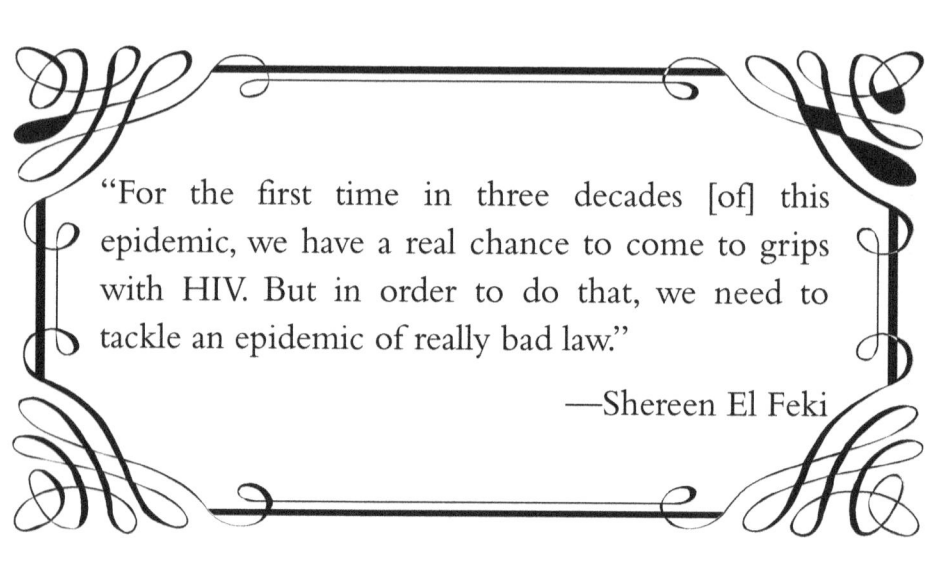

"For the first time in three decades [of] this epidemic, we have a real chance to come to grips with HIV. But in order to do that, we need to tackle an epidemic of really bad law."

—Shereen El Feki

PROPAGATED EPIDEMIC

Alhaji Omar was a very wealthy man with several companies and substantial shareholding in major multi-national companies in the country. With 12 children from his 4 wives, Alhaji's insatiable sexual appetite continues to make him prey on young girls in the neighbourhood.

Sometime in April, students of the State University began to notice the constant presence of Alhaji Omar on campus especially at odd hours of the night. Alhaji's new catch was Aisha the most "beautiful" student in the Department of Modern European Languages; tampered with by many, recycled by lecturers and loved by "gig" organizers.

As the relationship blossomed, Aisha made an unusual request, she asked Alhaji to divorce his first wife, the mother of 7 of his 12 children or consider the relationship over. Her request for the first wife to be divorced was tactical, as it will pave way for her to influence all his future decisions when she finally becomes his fourth wife.

Although a very difficult decision, Alhaji finally divorced his wife of 21 years for a lady whom he had come to love so much due to spiritual and herbal inducements.

The wedding ceremony was an elaborate one, which left students wondering how a highly depreciated Aisha got such a wealthy and influential man to marry her.

Not long after the wedding, Aisha who was already pregnant before the wedding started showing physical signs of pregnancy and was taken to the State Specialist Hospital to be registered at the antenatal clinic, it was at the clinic that the wind blew!—Aisha was

HIV positive and by this time Alhaji Omar and his other 3 wives, 2 of whom were nursing mothers were already carrying the virus.

Daily, thousands of innocent and faithful married women are infected with the HIV virus on their matrimonial beds. Some men consider the hunt for "sweet sixteen's" a civic responsibility and are ready to flirt with teens young enough to be their grandchildren, young girls on the other hand sit under their parents roofs to arrange flirting sessions with their father's peers using mobile gadgets bought by these terrorists. The activities of these men have reached a stage where young girls ages 11-16 now compete for the old man with the deepest pocket.

Nevertheless, when we fail to find the origin of a flashy or questionable item in a child's possession, we leave the door open for that child to spring up surprises that will have far reaching consequences.

Quote:

"We have lost our moral values and principles"
—Goodluck Jonathan

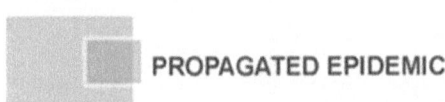

PROPAGATED EPIDEMIC

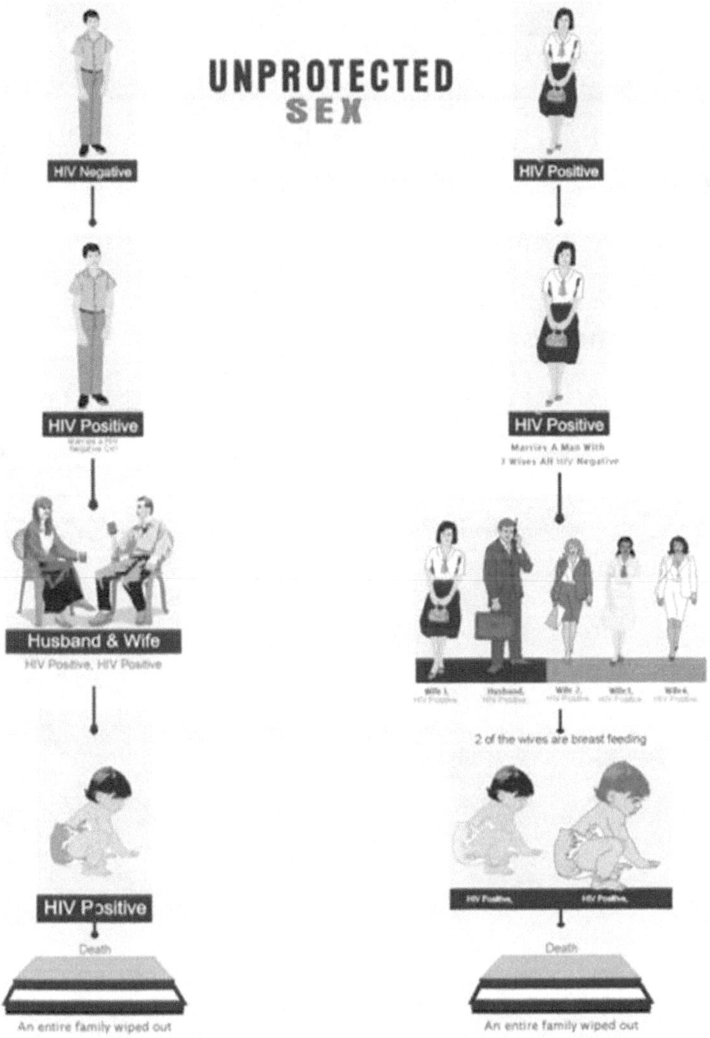

UNPROTECTED SEX

HIV Negative

HIV Positive
Marries a HIV
Negative Girl

Husband & Wife
HIV Positive, HIV Positive

HIV Positive

Death

An entire family wiped out

HIV Positive

HIV Positive
Marries A Man With
3 Wives All HIV Negative

Wife 1,
HIV Positive

Husband,
HIV Positive

Wife 2,
HIV Positive

Wife 3,
HIV Positive

Wife 4,
HIV Positive

2 of the wives are breast feeding

HIV Positive,

HIV Positive,

Death

An entire family wiped out

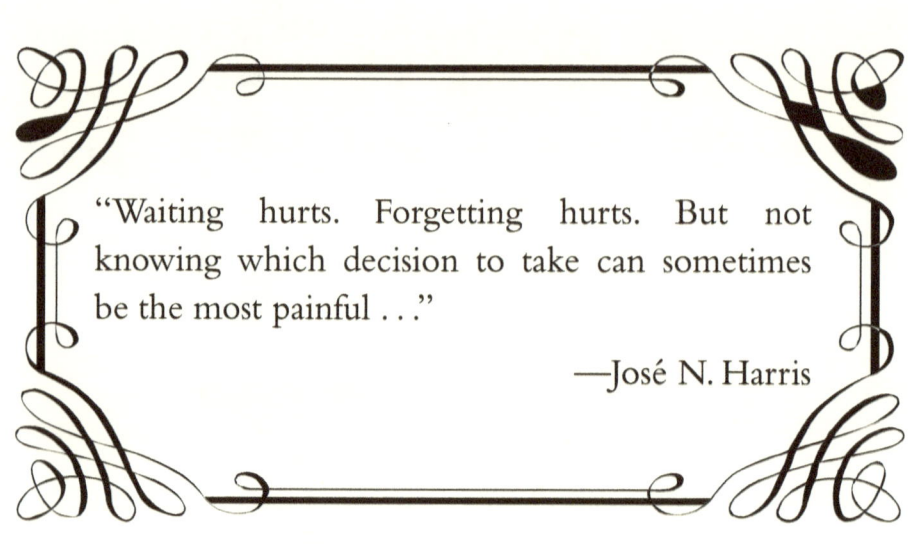

"Waiting hurts. Forgetting hurts. But not knowing which decision to take can sometimes be the most painful . . ."

—José N. Harris

NEGOTIATING SILENCE

Mrs. Umeh came to our small clinic in tears, her baby was dying, his body temperature was up and his arms and legs were twitching. She needed help and she wanted it fast.

As her cry for attention grew louder, I noticed a dark man about six and half feet tall trailing her everywhere she went.

Her child was looking malnourished and almost paper white. After consultation with the doctor, they were sent to the laboratory for urgent blood grouping as the child needed fresh blood transfusion. At the laboratory, the mystery man turned out to be the child's father, he had come to donate the blood his child needed.

As we carried out the required tests on his blood sample, it turned that Mr. Umeh, a police officer was HIV positive.

"Oga" he exclaimed please, please don't tell my wife, so we obtained the blood from another source after he made incoherent excuses to his wife on why he could not donate, and the child was transfused.

Few days later, after declining another post test counseling session, Mr. Umeh, appeared at my residence with a sack of beans and a white envelope in his hands. In his words "I have come to thank you for all the help and assistance you offered me and my wife when our child was on admission at your Hospital" As I watched him deceptively spew those words, he reminded me of his earlier demand that his test results be kept secret. I thankfully rejected his gifts and advised him to seek counsel and treatment fast.

As he left my house I realized how far people are willing to go in order to conceal an ailment.

Few months later, his wife was back at our clinic, this time to register at the antenatal clinic, I was interested in her HIV results and waited anxiously for it.

To the amazement of all including myself, the result was negative! I immediately asked for a repeat test and the result was the same, she was asked to return for another repeat test in 4 months time.

As I left the clinic that day, I pondered over many possibilities. As the disease control officer of the community, I was bent on ensuring that I had all the information before reaching a conclusion.

When she returned four months later, she was already seven months pregnant but was still looking strong and healthy. After her samples were collected and analyzed, the results still came back negative.

As she walked away with her results, the team brainstormed over the possibilities, as I was slid into depression. I knew Mr. Umeh had not been faithful to his wife, I knew he was HIV positive, I knew he did not want her to know, I knew I wanted to prevent her and her unborn child from getting infected, yet I was helpless because the tests were done in strict confidentiality.

Quote

"You can't make decisions based on fear and the possibility of what might happen."

—**Michelle Obama**

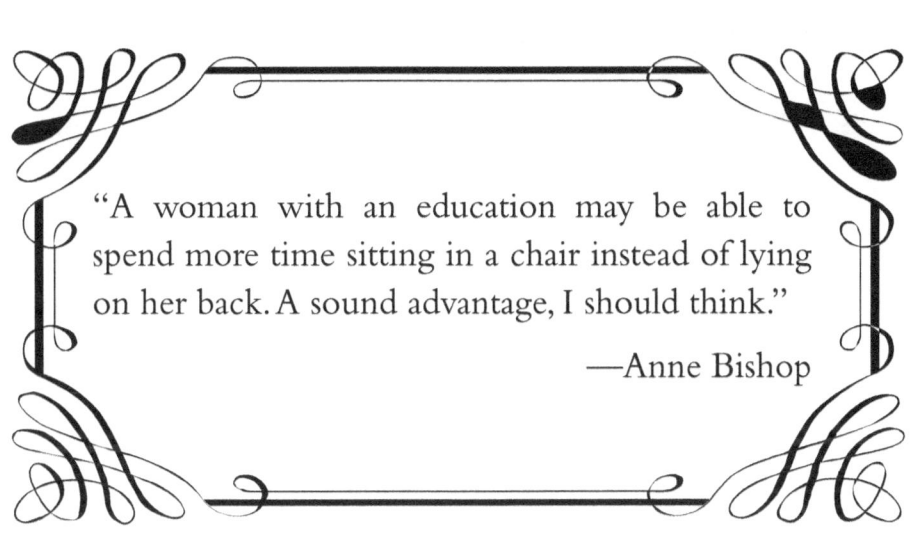

"A woman with an education may be able to spend more time sitting in a chair instead of lying on her back. A sound advantage, I should think."

—Anne Bishop

MONEY FOR HAND

"As a result of our findings from the laboratory report submitted to us which indicates that your wife to be is HIV positive, this Church is left with no other alternative but to call off the wedding" said the Pastor as a confused and perplexed Chuks sank deep into his seat completely lost in a state "*heebie jeebbie*"

Bro Chuks, a good looking and very hard working fellow went into a relationship with Sis Magdalene a retired commercial sex worker nick named "Money for hand" during her hey days, who is now a tongue speaking "born again" Christian.

Sis Magdalene who knew her positive status, began attending the Church earlier in the year after relocating from Kaduna, North West Nigeria to Abuja, Nigeria's capital city. In her quest to attract *Mr. Right*, she became very "spiritual" and was successful, before her luck ran out with the damning revelation of the contents of the laboratory result.

Her story is not different from Sarah Kabanda's, the fish monger from Kalangala district South of Uganda, who migrated to Kiruggu, concealed her identity and inflicted over 80 men who paid her for sex with the virus. The list is endless.

Our society has made it extremely difficult for those living with the virus to declare their status, perhaps if we were more accommodating, people like Magdalene and Sarah would have embraced the culture of positive living and educate others on ways to avoid been infected.

Advances in medical science have made it possible for a HIV negative individual to marry and have children with an infected partner and still remain uninfected.

With the expansion of the Prevention of Mother to Child Transmission (PMTCT) programme, infected mothers across the globe are increasingly giving birth to children devoid of the virus.

Successfully preventing mother to child transmission of HIV involves multiple layers of intervention, from pregnancy to child birth and extending to breastfeeding and other key components.

Although measuring the success rate of the prevention of mother to child programme is complicated, one thing is certain, it has been successful.

It is imperative for us to understand that being HIV positive is not a death sentence. The eradication of HIV/AIDS like any other disease will require a collective response.

Quote:

One way to be sure you are not making the wrong decision, is to look vertically upwards

—*Oche Otorkpa*

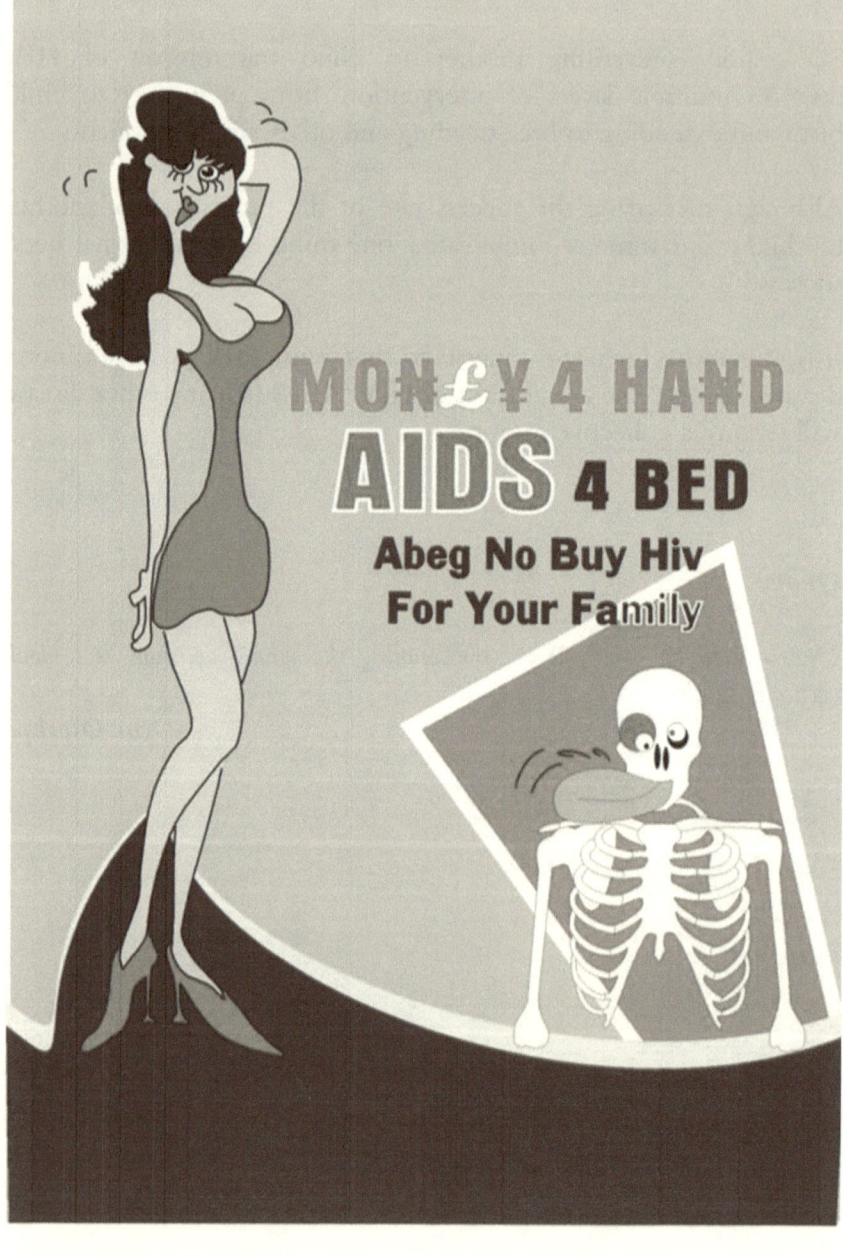

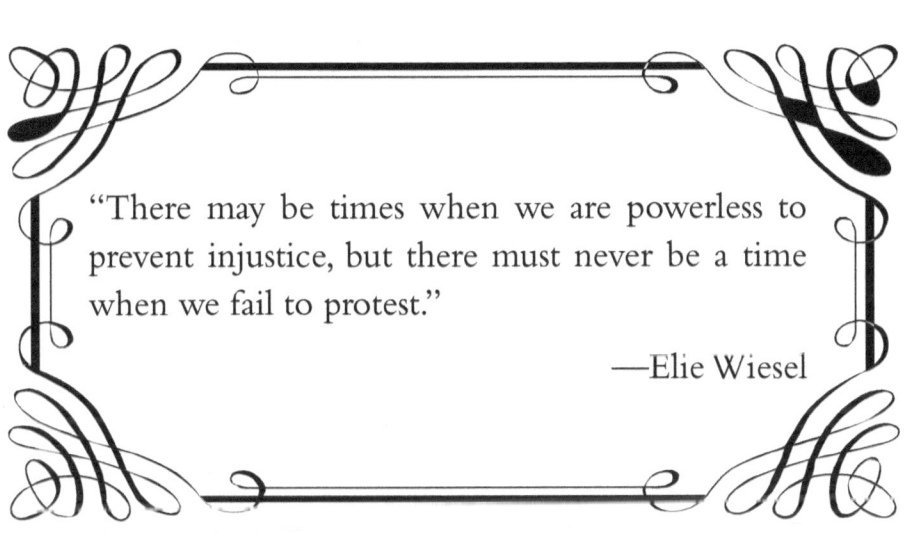

"There may be times when we are powerless to prevent injustice, but there must never be a time when we fail to protest."

—Elie Wiesel

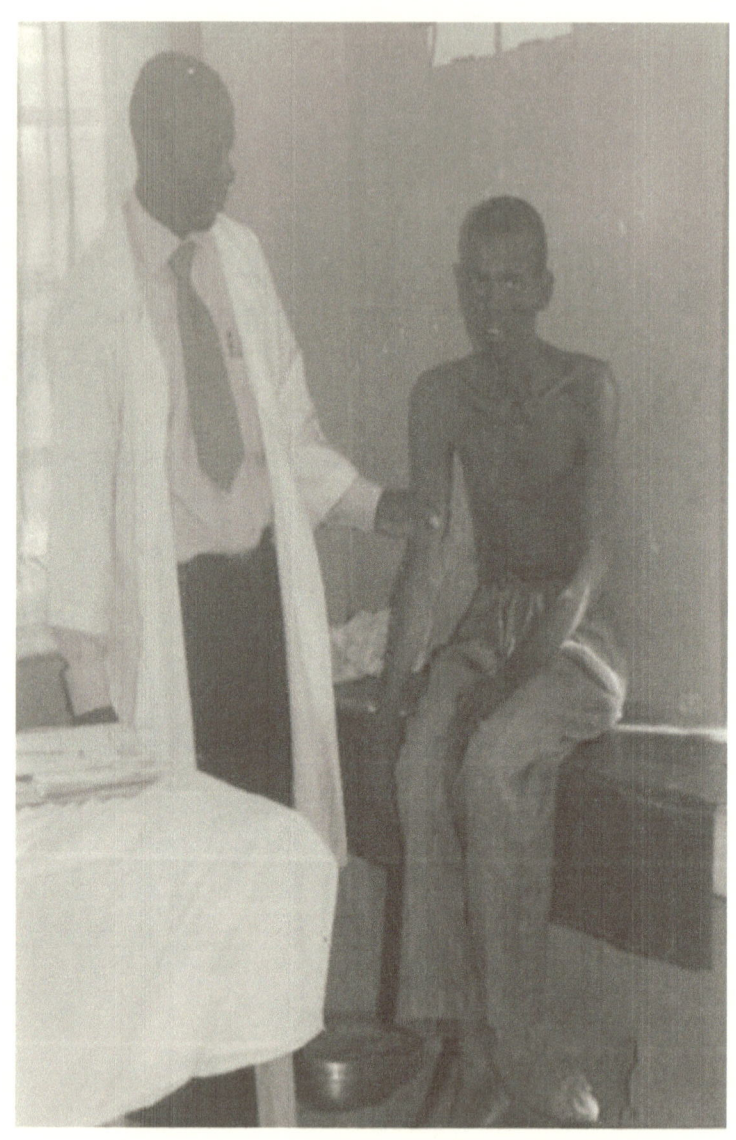

Helping abandoned AIDS patient's in rural Nigeria

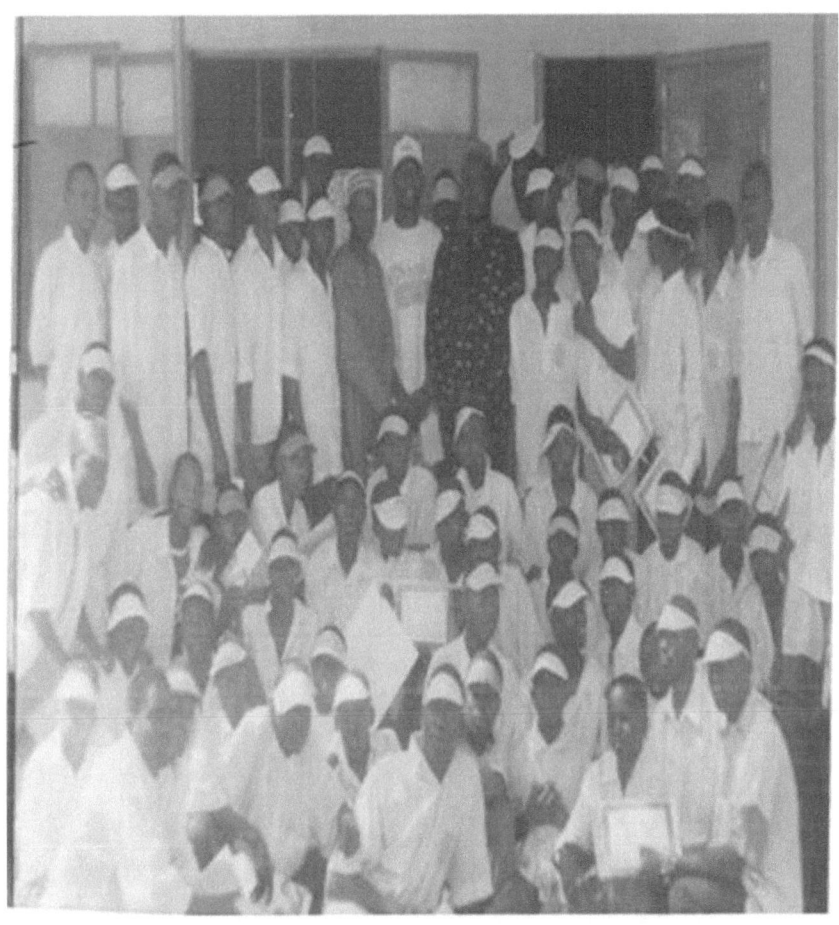

First set of Trainees for the UNICEF Supported Reproductive Health Training programme for Peer Educators at an all boys secondary school in Kurfi, Katsina State, Nigeria (2006)

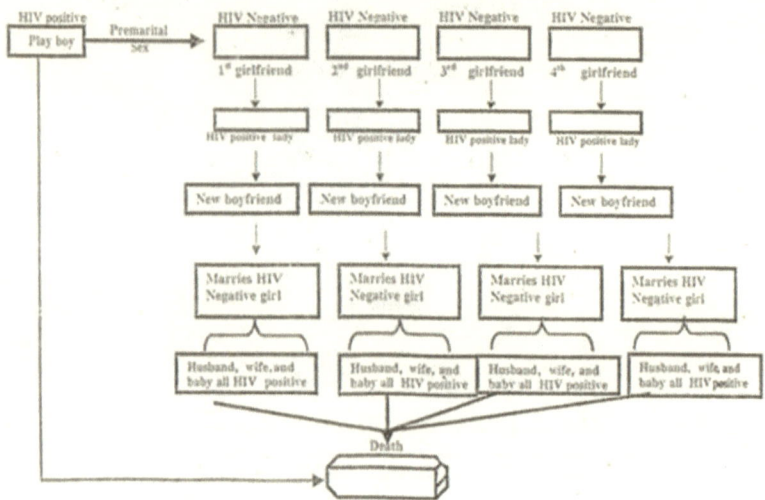

The original sketch of the playboy pathway designed by
Oche Otorkpa in 1999 for public Enlightenment

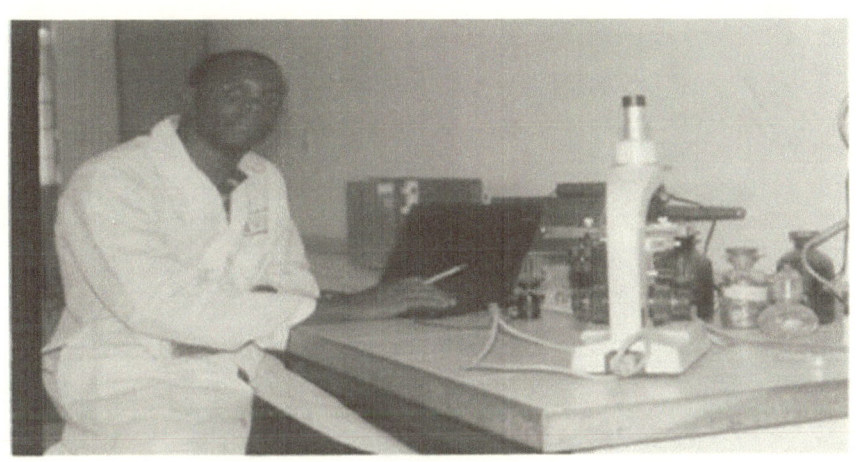

Oche at Microbiology laboratory in 2001.

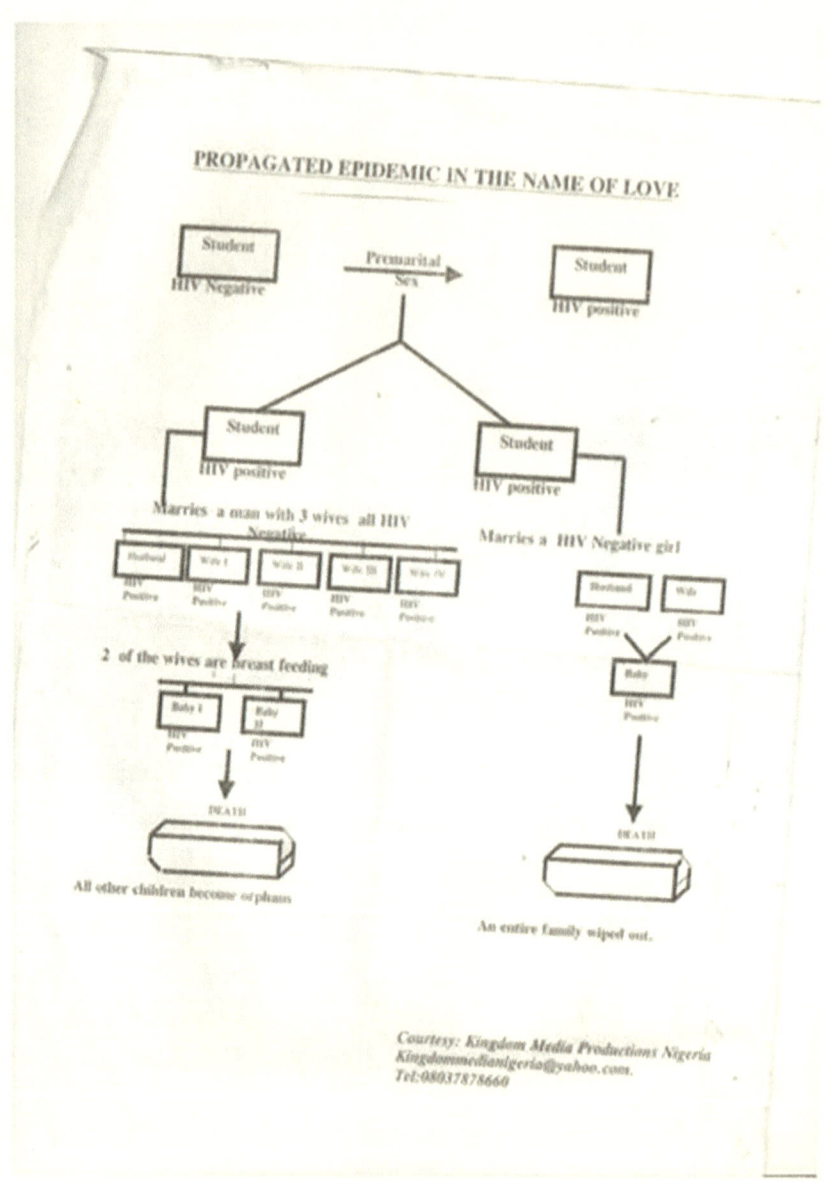

Original sketch of the propagated Epidemic pathway designed by Oche
Otorkpa in 2001

MONEY 4 HAND

AIDS

4 BED

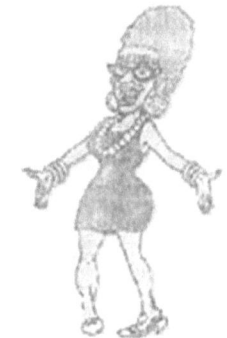

ABEG NO BUY HIV FOR YOUR FAMILY

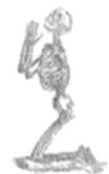

Original Enlightenment Campaign Material on Sex Trafficking Designed By Oche Otorkpa in 2004

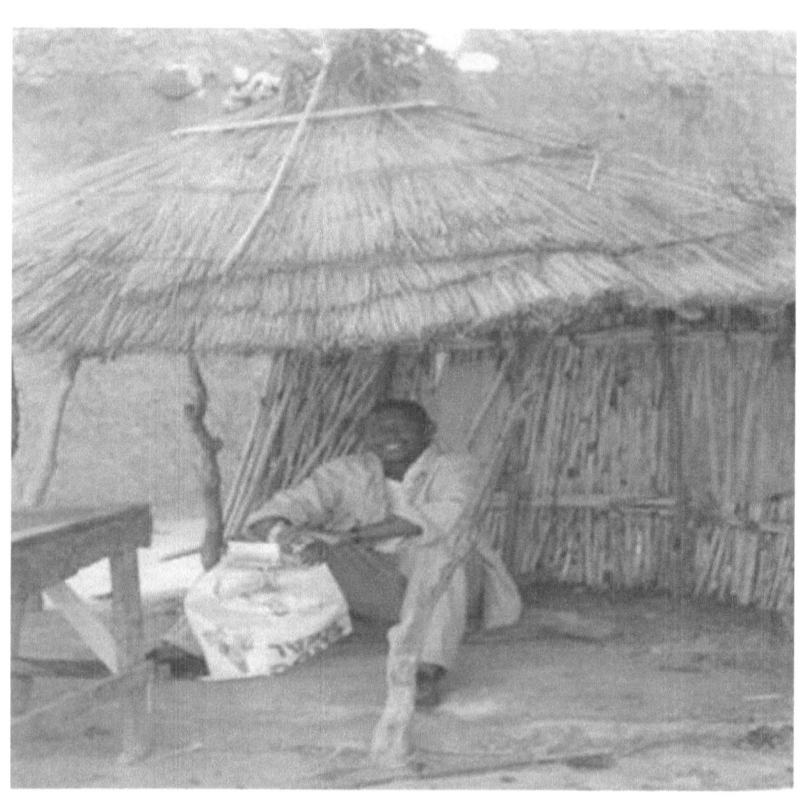

Oche at a village HIV enlightenment campaign in 2007

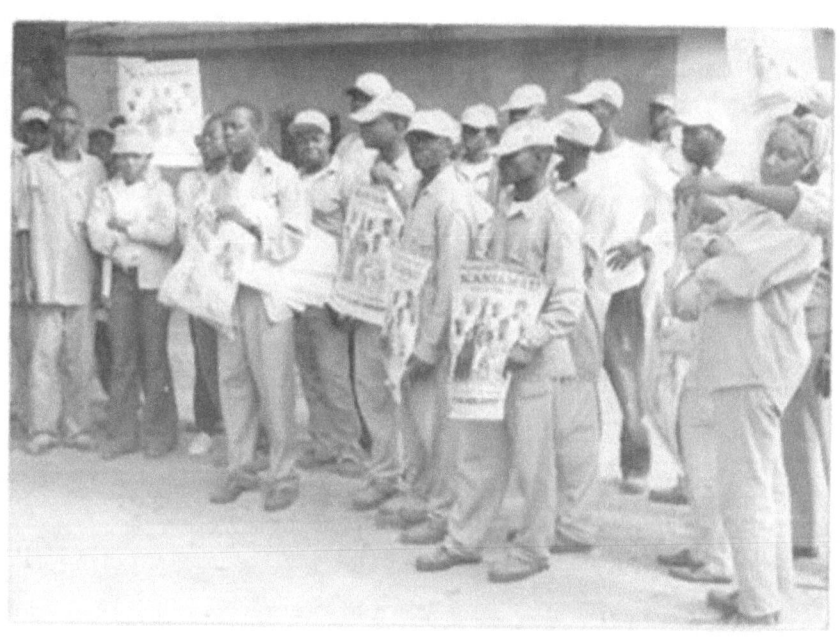

An Enlightenment campaign In Rawu Village North Western Nigeria

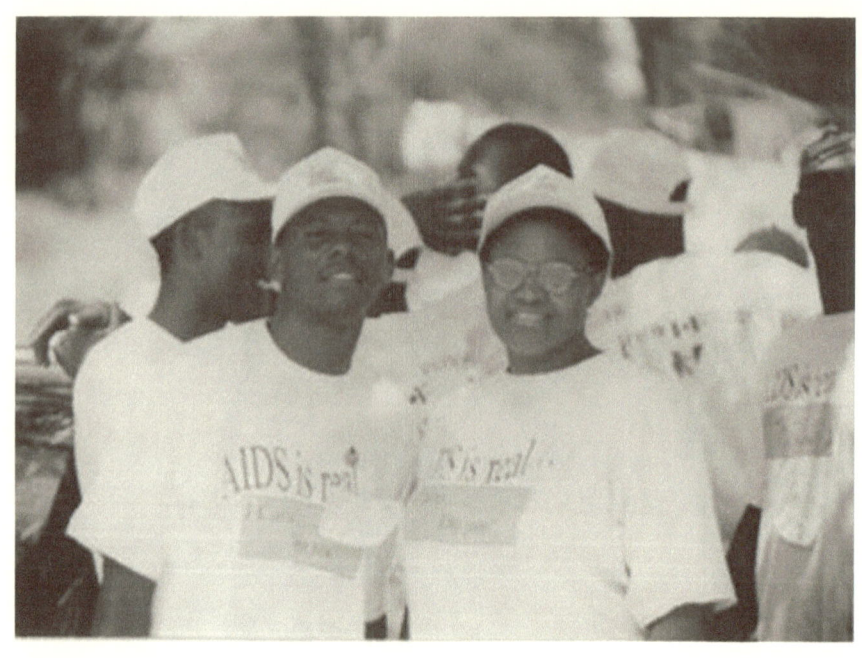

Oche With UNICEF's Dr Tinuke Omonayin at an event in 2006

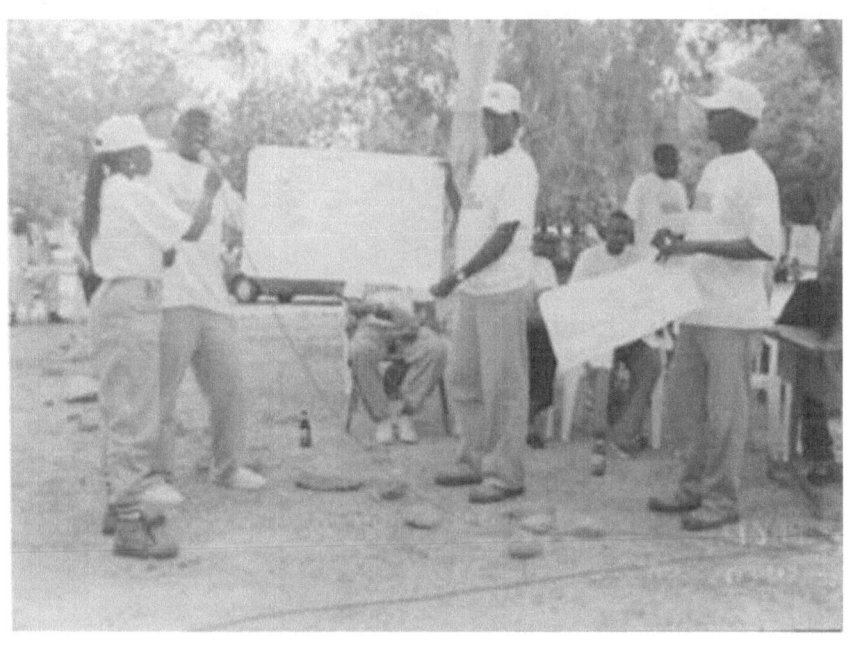

Passionately spreading the message at the National Youth Service Corps
Orientation camp in 2006

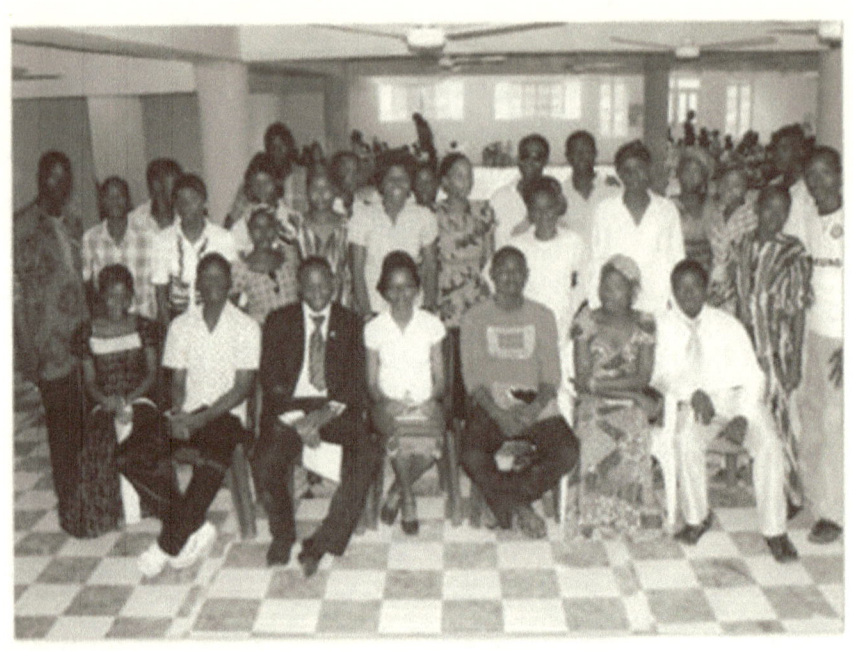

Empowering
Young people with the right information

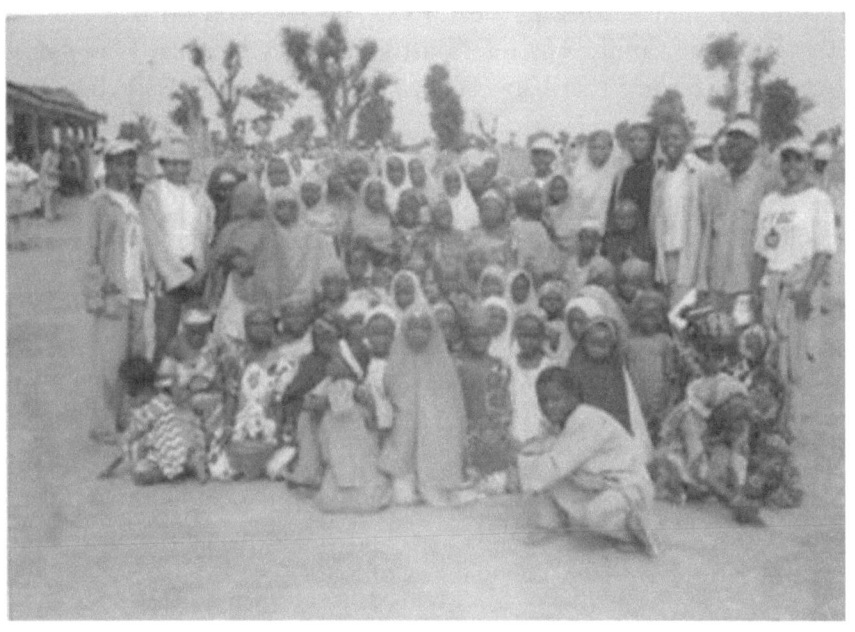

Equipping the younger Generation with the knowledge they need to secure the future

JUSTICE DENIED

Baby Hadiza had been in and out of the local clinic for the past six months. Born two years ago to a revered Islamic cleric in the village of Kida , Hadiza's health continued to deteriorate despite spending over 15 weeks on hospital admission and taking all the prescribed medications her health was still far from normal. Several days later, the family was referred to the city's General Hospital; it was at this facility that baby Hadiza was diagnosed with AIDS, but how? Protested the Cleric, looking visibly angry and emotionally distraught but that was it, his little girl was HIV positive. Subsequently, both parents were sent for HIV test but the results came out Negative.

However, going through the patient's medical records, the medical team soon realized that the baby was diagnosed with Anemia 12 months earlier and was transfused with 200mls of blood. Could this be the missing link?

Sharp practices and deliberate non compliance with standard procedures among health personnel especially in rural communities have led to several loss of lives.

In developing countries, corrupt politicians and contractors also tend to compound these problems with the supply of substandard equipments, fake reagents and outright embezzlement of funds appropriated for the development of health facilities in rural communities. To them and their co-conspirators, the pandemic is a money spinning machine that must be milked at all cost.

Endemic corruption has ensured that funds appropriated for HIV programmes end up in private bank accounts, leaving patients without medications and the public without kits to determine HIV status.

The presentation of claims for awareness programmes and events that never took place is perhaps the most worrying aspect of this kind of fraud, as it completely denies the public the critical information they would sometimes require in order to make lifestyle changes.

These activities coupled with the insensitivity and outright non compliance with standard procedures by some health workers has ensured that progress in the fight is consistently stagnated.

Today, the integrity of blood from blood banks in these areas remains a source of worry to many, while the locals have entrusted their lives to the hands of these few health professionals; some have betrayed that trust.

Quote

"Real integrity is doing the right thing, knowing that nobody's going to know whether you did it or not."

—Oprah Winfrey

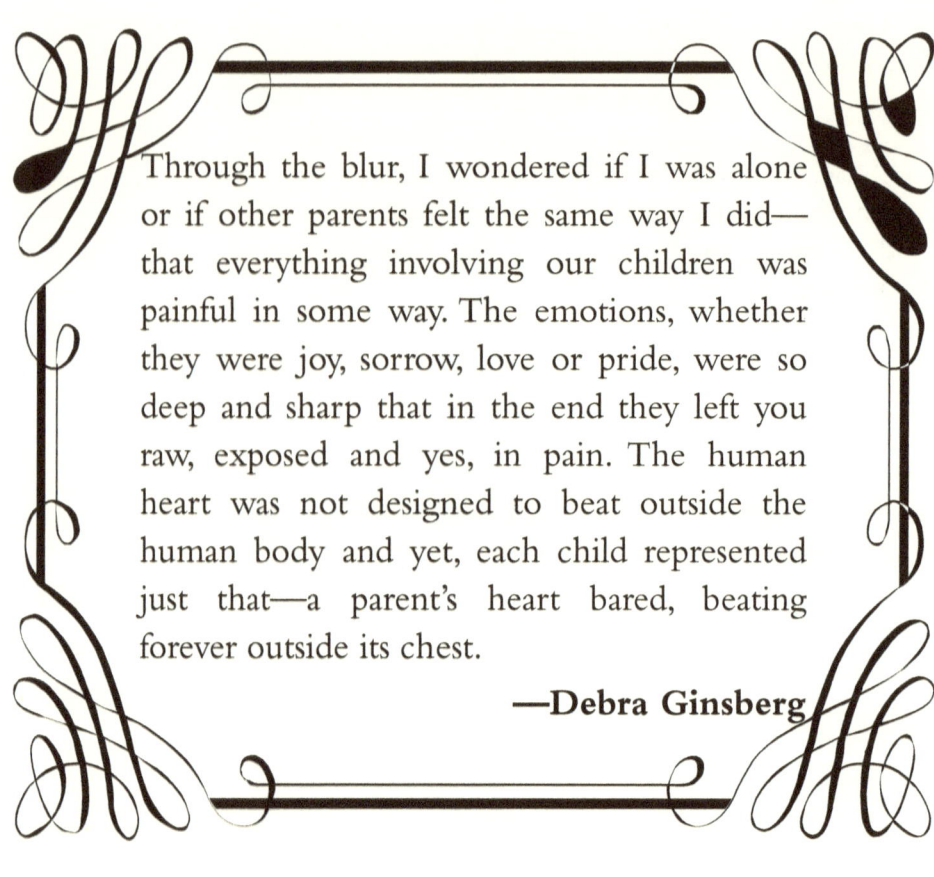

Through the blur, I wondered if I was alone or if other parents felt the same way I did—that everything involving our children was painful in some way. The emotions, whether they were joy, sorrow, love or pride, were so deep and sharp that in the end they left you raw, exposed and yes, in pain. The human heart was not designed to beat outside the human body and yet, each child represented just that—a parent's heart bared, beating forever outside its chest.

—**Debra Ginsberg**

THE PHONEBOOK

Debby has been having sex with Mr Offia her home lesson Teacher, since she was 10 and became pregnant for him at 14.

Neglected by her busy father and isolated by a mother who cares more about money making than raising kids, she sought solace in the arms of Mr Offia who consistently took advantage of her.

In her attempt to terminate the pregnancy using a local concoction, she fainted and was rushed to a hospital. At the hospital, she was diagnosed with acute liver failure due to the injection of poisonous substances; the doctor also informed her parents that she was carrying a child.

This unexpected turn of events triggered a series of "tsunamis" that altered the life of the family forever. As the doctors were battling to save her life, her situation got worse as she started bleeding from different orifice and lapsed into coma.

This prompted Debby's father to seek the intervention of law enforcement agents, who lunched a full scale investigation into the incident.

As they searched through her room, in a bid to find clues as to why the 14 year old will want to take her own life, they stumbled on an SMS sent to her mobile phone directing her on how to use a concoction to terminate the pregnancy.

However, the identity of the sender remained a mystery as the phone number saved as "My Chocolate" could not be traced to anyone.

While the police were trying to unravel the chocolate mystery, Debby's situation was getting worse, the occasional movement of fingers has not happened in three days and the family was becoming increasingly worried, while staff of the intensive care unit of the hospital continued to assure the family that they were doing all they could to ensure that their daughter pulls through.

After several days under the close watch of doctors and nurses, Debby eventually died, leaving her parents in a state of devastation.

As her corpse was been conveyed to the mortuary, the police invited her father for a chat, they have been analysing Debby's phone records and have discovered a pattern of calls made by a certain number registered to Mr Offia but saved as Mary on Debby's phonebook.

Mr Offia was eventually invited but he feigned ignorance of the abnormal phone book entry, stressing that his relationship with the deceased was purely academic, which manifested in her improved results at school, a claim he said could be substantiated by the deceased parents.

With no substantial evidence linking him to the death of the teenager, he was let off the hook and allowed to go home. But the police detectives believed he knew more than he was willing to admit, so they secured a search warrant and stormed his residence and to the relief of the team the search produced the "chocolate" sim card the police had been looking for as well as some of Debby's personal belongings.

Mr. Offia was later charged to court and is presently serving his sentence at a prison in Koton karfe, kogi state, Nigeria.

As I'm beginning to find out, parenting is no child's play, it could sometimes determine whether couples continue to live together or go their separate ways. No matter your temperament, your teenage child will drive you to the limit.

In my years as a teenage teacher and instructor, I have seen parents leave their homes so as to escape the torment and pain of trying to correct a teenage child.

The surging hormone makes it difficult for teenagers to view issues logically, making them increasing emotional. This is an aspect of teen development that is difficult to understand. Nevertheless, studies have shown that the frontal cortex of the Human brain does not develop until a person is within their twenties; the brain of a teenager is therefore a work in progress.

Building trust and openness is important if any relationship is to succeed. This also applies to the relationship between children and their parents, as children approach their teenage years, these surges in hormones and pressures from peers combine to make the teenage years the most challenging period for most parents.

Nevertheless, as I have discovered over the years, most parents tend to isolate a troubled teenager which further complicates an already difficult situation. Friendship, engagement and innovatively deploying activities that help teenagers channel their energy and redirect their anger are some of the pathways that have helped several parents find the rhythm in their quest to achieve a balanced relationship with their children.

A complex world of intrigues and power play among couples has combined to deny young people the love and attention they truly deserve, more and more teenagers are leaving home to peer up with bad influence which eventually lands them in jail for the lucky ones and six feet under for the not so lucky.

The Media and the internet have taken up the responsibility of moulding the young ones amongst us, leaving us to pursue the careers we treasure. But in the end we will all pay the price for the moral mistake we all combine to initiate and live with the repercussions of raising a generation without values.

Directly or indirectly, we owe these kids the responsibility of letting them know that they are loved, and that despite the barrage of challenges they face in a world that is constantly changing, we will never turn our backs on them.

Quote.

We may not be able to prepare the future of our children, but we can at least prepare our children for the future

—**Franklin D. Roosevelt**

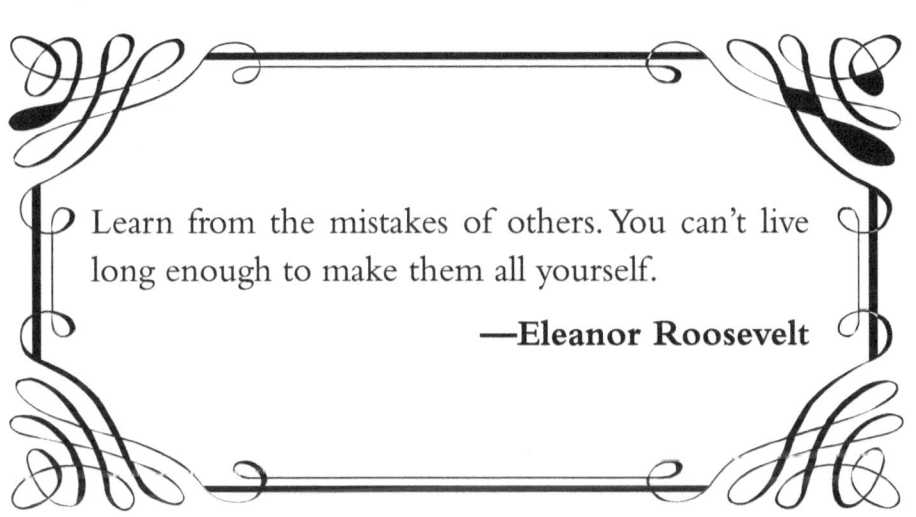

Learn from the mistakes of others. You can't live long enough to make them all yourself.

—**Eleanor Roosevelt**

RIVER BENUE

Lance corporal Idibia arrived the Murtala Mohammed International Airport in high spirits, he had been part of the United Nations Peace keeping contingent to the Sudanese region of Darfur. He and his colleagues had just been relieved by another battalion after spending close to a year under the harsh climatic conditions of the area, where waves of dust and regular whirlwinds were a normal occurrence.

Top on Idibia's mind on arrival, was how to find the wife of his dreams, his 35th birthday was approaching and he knew it was time to settle down, but there was a problem, he wanted a girl with good moral upbringing, untainted by the greed and immorality that comes with city life. As a soldier, he was known for his up rightness and high moral standards and he concluded that the city was not a place to find one.

On a trip to Oturkpo his home town, he shared his burden with Maria his elder sister who suggested Ochanya, the daughter of the village priest, she was the poster girl for chastity in the village. He accepted her recommendation and sought the family's approval to marry their daughter.

On his next visit, a wedding date was fixed, and few weeks later the wedding took place to the delight of both families and Idibia returned to the battalion with his new bride Ochanya. Nine months later, Ochanya gave birth to a baby boy to the delight of her Husband and the family was doing quite well.

Trouble started when the child fell sick and hospital visits became regular. At 20 months old the child was diagnosed with AIDS, Mr Idibia was stunned! He knew he tested Negative on return from peace keeping mission, and never had any sexual relationship with anyone outside marriage! How could his child be HIV positive he argued. He and his wife were later screened and the results came back positive.

Shocked and enraged Idibia confronted his wife who feigned ignorance of how the family came about the Infection.

As the controversy raged on, an enlarged family meeting was summoned by the village head with both families in attendance. However, the meeting ended in a stalemate as both families pointed accusing fingers at each other.

The controversy was not resolved, until Ochanya opened up to her mother on her death bed, she told her that on the day before Idibia came to ask for her hand in marriage, she had sex for the very first time with Ogaba the village church choirmaster who died of AIDS six months earlier, with tears rolling down her eyes, she pleaded with her mum to forgive her, as she lay helpless on her hospital bed coughing intermittently.

I come from Benue state, North central Nigeria where the virus continues to ravage many communities, not because governments have not intervened but because our people have refused to change the lifestyle that brought us to this pitiable state, our actions has ensured that we made headlines for all the wrong reasons.

Sadly, many others have copied our dangerous lifestyle which has transformed farmers who previously cultivate large hectares of farmland to paupers. With sky rocketing rates of teenage pregnancy and alcohol induced suicidal behaviours, the world expects more from a state that prides itself as the food basket of the nation.

Quote

I alone cannot change the world, but I can cast a stone across the waters to create many ripples.

—**Mother Teresa**

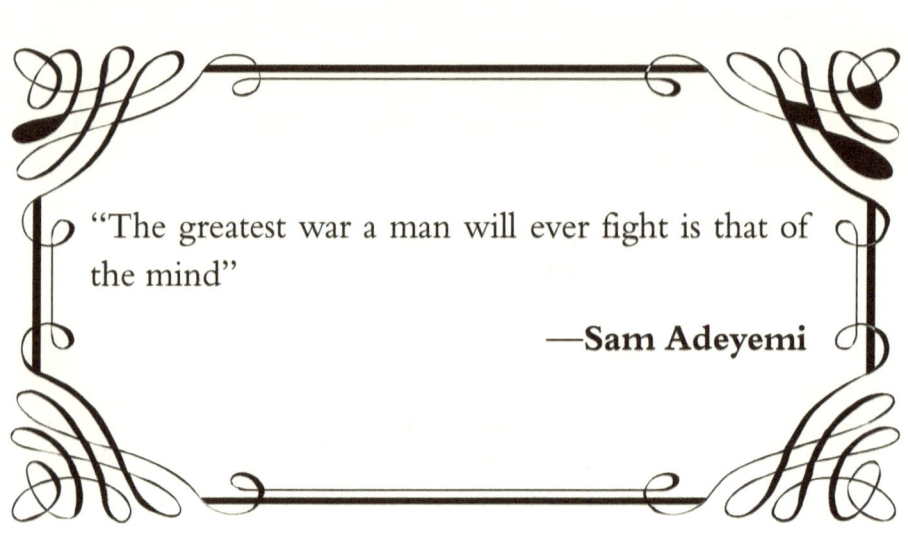

"The greatest war a man will ever fight is that of the mind"

—**Sam Adeyemi**

MR. LECTURER

A = Belongs to God
B = Belongs to me
C = Is for the very few best students
D = Is for the average students
E = Is for Everybody.
F = Is for those who question this decree.

This is the Gospel according to Dr. Noah, a randy lecturer in one of the Universities in South Eastern Nigeria. It is on record that beautiful girls in any class he lectures always have problems with their continuous assessment (C.A) and as such must "see him".

Few days before the commencement of the second semester examinations, news filtered into the campus that Mr. Lecturer is now HIV positive and was placed on antiretroviral drugs 2 weeks earlier. This shocking news elicited wild celebration among students in a lecture hall who saw the lecturer's condition as an end to his reign of terror, but one particular event did not go unnoticed, some female students left the hall panicking with tears almost rolling down their cheeks. You don't need Google to find reasons for such show of deep emotions, it's payback time for those who were awarded A and B grades for deliberately missing lectures and course tests, the fear that they might have contracted the virus during the one-on-one lecture series has become a great source of concern.

But why have some students' chosen to trade their bodies for grades?

While HIV silently kills more students than cultists and gangsters combined, it continues to receive less attention from school administrators. The word HIV has become a taboo word for some lecturers and teachers who are guilty of compromising their office for pleasure.

Perhaps, those charged with the responsibility of imparting knowledge and promoting good conduct have slipped into amnesia and need to be reminded of their responsibilities.

If lecturers and tutors can dedicate a minimum of 20 minutes once every semester or session for lectures, debates or discussions among their students on the threat posed by the pandemic may be their students might just take a cue.

Quote:

"Spread the Knowledge, not the Virus"

—Oche Otorkpa

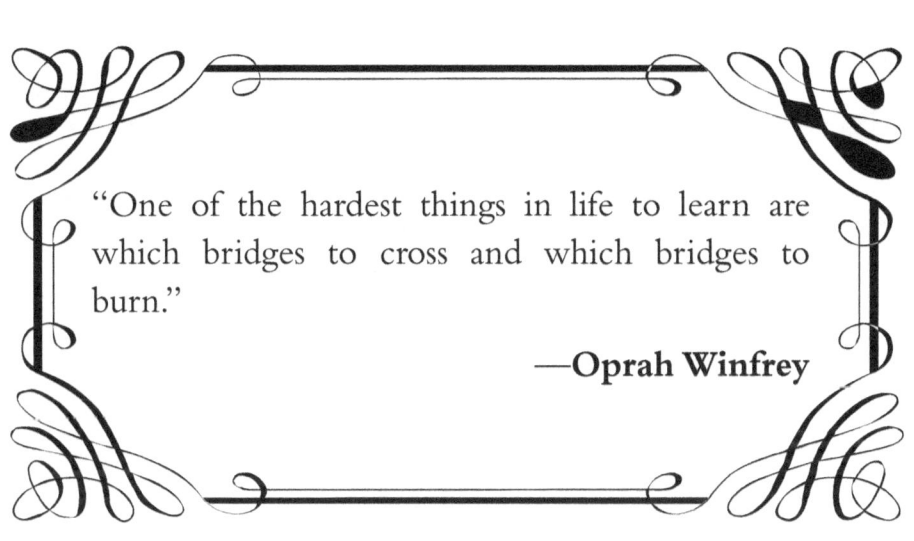

"One of the hardest things in life to learn are which bridges to cross and which bridges to burn."

—**Oprah Winfrey**

MY STORY

My name is Hadiza, I am 30 years old and a Graduate of computer science from the Bayero University Kano, North west Nigeria. I decided to tell my own story because I felt the burden on my shoulders will only be lifted when I let others know what I put myself through.

Few years ago, I was engaged to be married to Bashir the son of my Father's Best friend Alhaji Tanko. We had grown up together so I knew him quite well.

All was going on well until I attended Rukkaya's 20th Birthday Party. It was at that event I was introduced to Shehu, a good looking Insurance Executive who was working in Katsina at that time.

After that meeting, we exchanged few visits and the relationship blossomed despite protests from Bashir my fiancé.

Shehu was a man who could make any woman laugh, I enjoyed his company and felt nothing could ever separate us. As our relationship advanced, my behavior towards Bashir changed completely and all attempts by friends and family members to settle the rift tore us further apart, not even my father could make me change my mind as my heart was fixed. Bashir was heartbroken but I had moved on.

One day, while going through Shehu's mobile phone I realized I had made the biggest mistake of my entire life, Shehu was a Snake! Unknown to Rukkaya my friend and Bilkisu my classmate Shehu was dating the three of us simultaneously including other girls we did not know.

When I confronted Shehu, he flared up and gave me the beating of my life. Faced with the reality that I have burnt all my bridges,

I returned to the hostel the following day, treated my wounds and moved on with life as if nothing happened.

13 months later, I graduated with a second class upper degree and by this time Bashir had married my cousin Zaliha and they were expecting their first child.

During the Worlds AIDS Day, five years ago I accidentally came across an organization conducting free voluntary confidential counseling and testing. I decided to screen myself, that was when I discovered that I was carrying the virus.

It's Been 5 years now, and every day I wake up I just can't seem to forgive myself, the agony of taking drugs for the rest of my Life seem too much for me to bear.

As I open the container of Anti retroviral drugs every morning and evening I am constantly reminded that we are a products of the choices we make.

Quote:

"I am not a saint, unless you think of a saint as a sinner who keeps on trying."

—Nelson Mandela

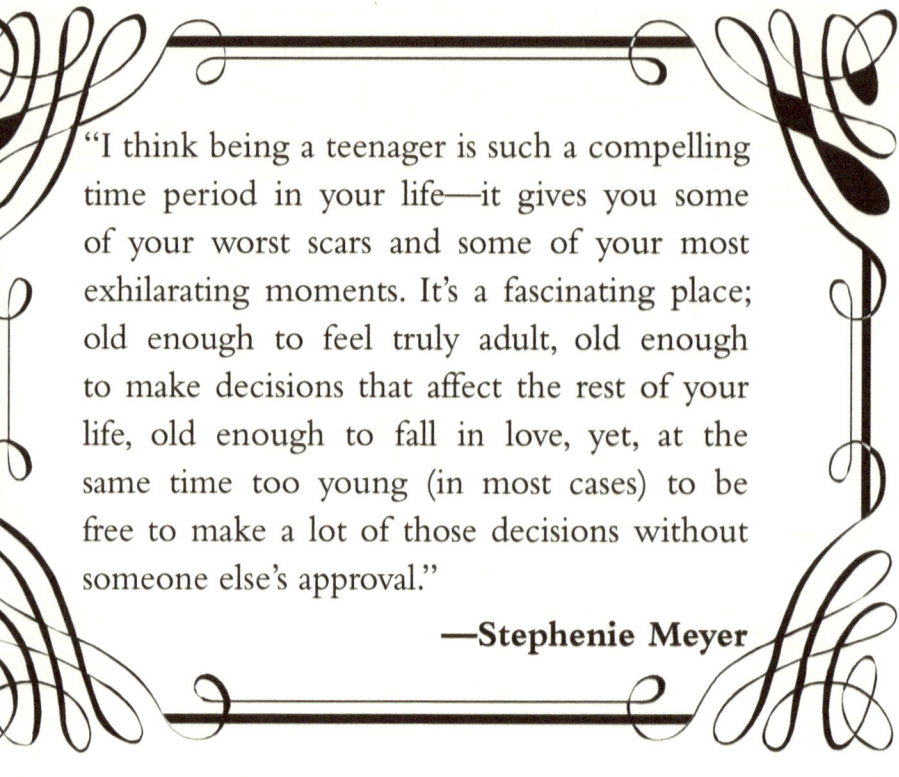

"I think being a teenager is such a compelling time period in your life—it gives you some of your worst scars and some of your most exhilarating moments. It's a fascinating place; old enough to feel truly adult, old enough to make decisions that affect the rest of your life, old enough to fall in love, yet, at the same time too young (in most cases) to be free to make a lot of those decisions without someone else's approval."

—Stephenie Meyer

HORMONE KINETICS

Few months to my Senior Secondary School Leaving Certificate Examination (SSCE) my landlady issued me a sudden quit notice four months ahead of my next due date for payment, the old lady would have none of my pleas as she handed me the one week notice. Her son was returning from the United States and she needed to renovate the apartment for him to occupy.

I have been living alone since my family moved to Abuja. My dad was transferred to the Supreme Court and I needed to complete my senior secondary school (high school) before joining them. Confused and perplexed I dressed up and headed for school, as I approached the School gate I suddenly realized that in the midst of the confusion I had left my school bag at home, such was my state of mind as entered the classroom.

I spent 9 days living in an abandoned car, sneaking in at night and rising up early to avoid any suspicion all in a bid to tell the world am old enough to take care of myself. During that period, I spoke to my father several times using the public phone booth without letting him know his Son was a homeless student. One night, as I lay on a mat inside the abandoned car, I could hear the cry of a young girl been molested by hoodlums, as her cry echoed through the darkness I realized I had taken a decision that could potentially cost me my life.

With mosquitoes having filled nights draining blood from my veins, and the bark of several rabies infected stray dogs interrupting my sleep for nine days, I gave up and sought for help.

The sudden surge of hormones at teenage age will continue to play an important part in the life of young people. As they struggle to come to terms with their emerging sexuality, many will make decisions that could significantly alter their lives forever.

So many interests compete for our young people, from drug barons to sex traffickers who are constantly looking for ways to revive their ageing workforce by perpetually enslaving these young minds. These recruitment schemes have polluted the blood lines in many communities transforming promising young men and women into lawful captives.

One of the greatest challenge facing young people today, is the large scale availability of half truth's and manipulated facts. If young people are our greatest asset in a war that must be won then we must be willing to extricate them at whatever cost from the clutches of those who seek to exploit their weaknesses and constructively engage them in the conceptualization and formulation of policies and programmes geared towards influencing behavioral patterns in the society.

Quote

Shoving policies and programmes down the throats to young people has never worked and never will

—**Oche Otorkpa**

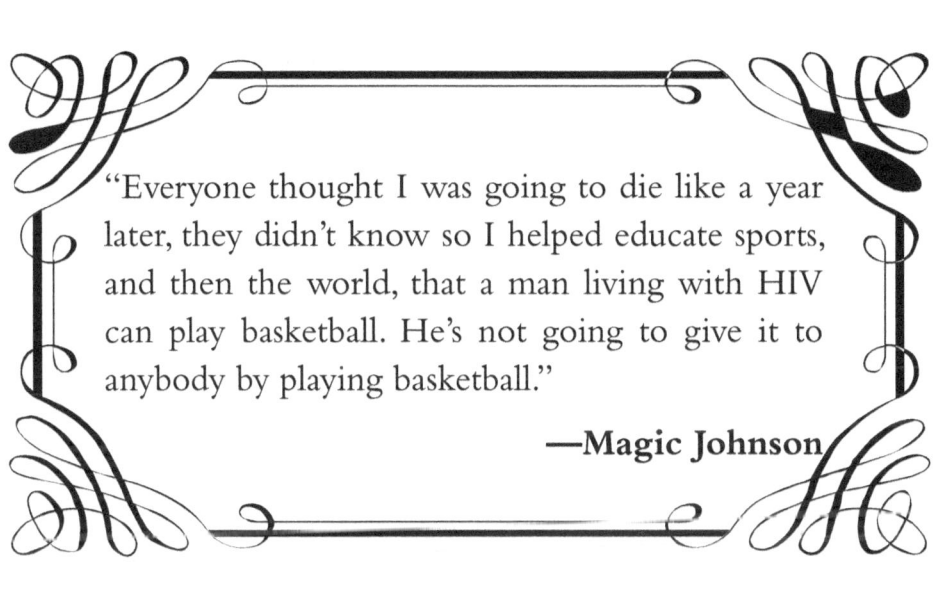

"Everyone thought I was going to die like a year later, they didn't know so I helped educate sports, and then the world, that a man living with HIV can play basketball. He's not going to give it to anybody by playing basketball."

—**Magic Johnson**

SUPPORTIVELY CARING

Imabong committed suicide because of the rejection she suffered as a result of her HIV status; isolated by her family, rejected by her friends and treated like a leper at work was more than she could bear.

When I met Luke in February of 2007, he had not eaten for 2 days; dehydrated and completely emaciated, he could barely utter a word. Abandoned to his fate in a one room apartment, Luke prayed for death but it never came.

The commercial drivers he recruited to run his small transport business moved to other cities with his buses leaving him with almost nothing.

As humanity confronts the AIDS pandemic stigmatization, misery and isolation appears to have taken centre stage. While it is true that about 90% of HIV infection occur via the sexual route this must never be misconstrued for promiscuity. It is wrong to ascribe promiscuity to a woman who got infected on her matrimonial bed, a victim of rape who tested positive, or a victim of HIV infected blood transfusion. These people need love to overcome the fear, anger and regret. They need our care and support to move on with life.

The stigmatization and the excruciating pains of social alienation have compelled most victims to conceal their status while the malevolent ones continue to distribute the virus free of charge to unsuspecting men and women.

We must be willing to change our attitude towards people living with the virus if we are to make any meaningful progress in curtailing the spread of the disease. If most of us won't seat on the same couch with someone who is infected, how do we expect other carriers to declare their status? Our perceptions notwithstanding, these people are still part of us and won't disappear.

A planet without AIDS is possible, but to create that planet we must do away with the vestiges of the old planet where testing positive to the HIV virus effectively relegates an individual to the subclass of Human society.

Albert Einstein defined insanity as doing the same thing over and over but expecting a different result, we therefore need a new direction if we must make any progress.

While we must be bold enough to confront the ills in the society that promotes the spread of the disease, we must also remember that we ourselves are not perfect either.

Quote:

"HIV does not make people dangerous to know, so you can shake their hands and give them a hug: Heaven knows they need it"

—Princess Diana

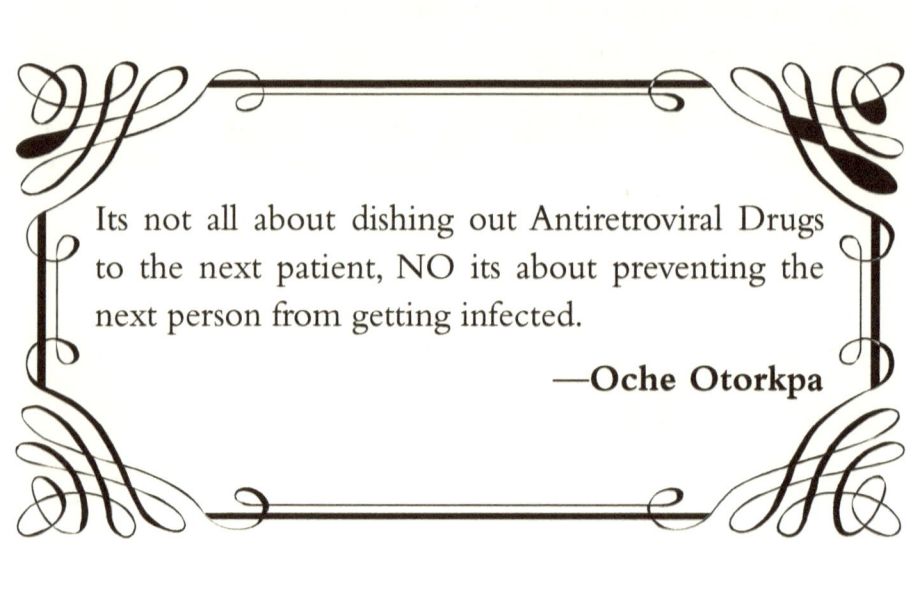

Its not all about dishing out Antiretroviral Drugs to the next patient, NO its about preventing the next person from getting infected.

—Oche Otorkpa

WELCOME TO
THE CLINIC

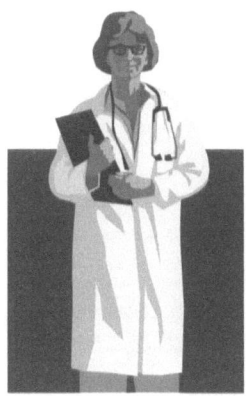

What is HIV?

HIV stands for "Human Immuno Deficiency Virus" it is the causative agent of AIDS.

What is AIDS?

AIDS stands for "Acquired Immune Deficiency Syndrome". It is caused by the HIV virus which weakens the immune System (body's defence mechanism) and makes a person susceptible to all kinds of infections.

How is HIV Transmitted?

HIV can be contracted by the following ways:

> ➢ During sexual intercourse with an infected person (vaginal, oral and anal).

> ➢ During transfusion of an infected blood

> ➢ By the use of contaminated and unsterilized sharp instruments such as syringes.

➢ From infected mother to child during pregnancy, child birth or breast feeding.

How is HIV not transmitted?

HIV cannot be transmitted by

➢ Mosquito bites

➢ Handshake with an infected person

➢ Cloths

➢ Sharing toilet seats with an infected person

➢ Hugging an infected person

➢ Eating or playing with an infected person

HIV and mosquitoes

For an infectious agent to be transmitted by a mosquito from one person to another, it must remain viable inside the mosquito. This is however not true for the AIDS virus as the mosquitoes treats the virus as food which is digested along with the blood meal. 70 to 80% of HIV infected persons have undetectable virus particles in their blood. Calculations have shown that a mosquito that is interrupted while feeding on a HIV carrier circulating 1000 units of virus has a 1: 10 million probability of injecting a single unit to an HIV free recipient, that is to say an individual has to be bitten by 10million mosquitoes that has began feeding on a HIV carrier to be infected.

Furthermore, the mechanism utilised by mosquitoes during feeding differs greatly from the mechanism employed by the drug user's needle. This is because it delivers salivary fluid through one passage and draw blood up another as such the food canal is not flushed like a used needle and blood flow is unidirectional. In simple language mosquitoes do not transmit HIV.

HIV and Kissing

Although the risk of transmission is very low, the presence of sores or abrasions on the mouth could make that "simple kiss" deadly. This is because the virus is present in all body fluids although in varying concentration.

Diagnosis

This is usually carried out using immunochromatographic strips which determines the presence of the antibodies in the bloodstream (ELISA). This test is usually confidential and often requires the consent of the individual after proper counselling.

Other methods include western blot and the use of the PCR machine.

Signs and Symptoms

When an individual is infected with the virus that does not imply that he or she has AIDS. The individual is simply HIV infected. AIDS which is the final stage of the infection has the following symptoms.

1. Prolong diarrhoea

2. Oral thrush

3. Lymph gland enlargement

4. Persistent fever

5. Persistent cough

6. Skin infections

7. Unexplained weight loss

Phases

There are four phases of the infections,

Window period: This could last for about 3-6 months after exposure to the virus. During this period laboratory diagnosis often appear negative.

Healthy stage: During this period an individual appears healthy and may remain so for 3-10 years this is however dependant on nutrition and lifestyle.

Unhealthy stage: During this period the individual fall sick very often as the virus weakens the immune system.

Full blown AIDS: This is the final stage of the infection. It has duration of 12-24 months.

Prevention

The best and safest means of preventing HIV infection is ABSTINENCE from sexual intercourse for unmarried people and FAITHFULNESS among married couples.

Condom and HIV

Some researchers have argued that condoms do not prevent the transmission of HIV. Their argument is based on the size of the virus. They argue that because of the minute size of the virus (0.1 microns or 4 billionth of an inch) it could easily pass through the pores of the condom which is about 450 microns in size.

On the other hand, most researchers agree that since the virus is transmitted via a medium which cannot breach the integrity of the condom then condoms do prevent HIV transmission. Nevertheless, it is generally agreed that a ruptured or leaking condom is a health risk that those who belong to the famous "I no fit hold body" club must face.

Whichever side of the divide you belong, it is advised that you fully explore the option of abstinence which is the safest means of prevention before resorting to condoms.

Microbicides

These are substances that will be available as creams, gels, films, suppositories or vaginal rings, which if applied vaginally have the ability to reduce the risk of HIV and STIs transmission during sexual intercourse. Some microbicides under development can also act as spermicide which kills sperm cells providing a relative contraceptive cover in the process.

Treatment and Cure

As a cure for AIDS continues to elude Scientists, Antiretroviral drugs continue to play a very important role in the treatment of AIDS patients, reducing the viral load and making treatment for opportunistic infections less complicated.

Despite claims both locally and internationally, a curative therapy does not appear to be in sight. However, the Pugnacious claim that sex with virgins can cure AIDS is the greatest deception of the 21st century.

WHAT TO DO WHEN YOU ARE NOT SURE OF YOUR HIV STATUS

Globally 9 out ten infected people do not know they carry the virus, this is disturbing because early detection in most cases is the difference between life and death.

The first question an individual must ask his or her self is:

➢ **What is my HIV status?**

➢ **If my previous status was negative, have I engaged in any risky behaviour that could compromise my initial status?**

Nearly everyone I know was afraid of the outcome on their first HIV test result, so if you are feeling scared, it is completely normal and not out of place. Knowing your HIV status is very important as it helps you to make the correct decisions about your life.

Another critical question is—**When should I get tested?**

Most people get tested for the very first time when they are about to get married, this is wrong! There is no guarantee that the results that came back negative before the wedding will not change after the six months window period. It's important for partners willing to pursue a relationship to discuss their HIV status before committing to the relationship.

Regular testing is a necessity for individuals having unprotected sex and for persons with multiple sexual partners.

So when you are not sure of your HIV status, the most intelligent thing to do is to walk into a testing centre and get yourself tested.

WHAT TO DO WHEN YOUR TEST RESULT IS POSITIVE

A HIV positive test result is not a death sentence, many HIV carriers are alive and doing very well decades after they tested positive. Advances in medical science has ensured that HIV positive individuals live a normal life as much as possible.

Most test centres have trained and qualified counsellors who will guide the individual on appropriate lifestyle changes to make where necessary.

Networking among HIV positive individuals have been shown to positively affect the lives of HIV carriers, these networking programmes have not only improved the quality of life among people living with HIV, it has also boosted self determination and personal development of people living with the virus.

Therefore getting involved with the activities of these groups will be highly beneficial to anyone who tested positive.

Taking drastic decision after testing positive can have devastating effects; it is therefore advised that persons who tested positive seek counsel before making major lifestyle changes.

WHAT TO DO WHEN YOUR TEST RESULT IS NEGATIVE

When the result of a HIV test is negative, it is usually advised that the individual returns after some months for a repeat test. A repeat test is carried out to confirm the result of the initial test.

The period between infection and the detection of antibodies within the blood stream is usually referred to as the Window period. During this period antibodies against the HIV virus are not detectable as such the test are usually negative.

A negative result after a confirmatory test does not mean the individual is immune to the virus, it only confirms the fact that the individual is not infected with the virus.

Persons who tested negative should note that, it is their responsibility to ensure that they remain negative, as allowing any slip could be deadly. To remain negative you will find the following steps helpful

- ➢ Avoid unprotected sex (Vaginal, Oral or Anal)

- ➢ Avoid multiple sexual partners

- ➢ Avoid injecting drug and illicit substances

- ➢ Avoid contaminated sharp objects

- ➢ Stay faithful to your partner

- ➢ Go for medical check up regularly

- ➢ Discuss HIV before committing to a relationship

- ➢ Seek counsel whenever in doubt about any issue.

Any information at your disposal that is not used is useless; it is our collective responsibility to ensure an AIDS free world.

Quote:

We all do better when we work together. Our differences do matter, but our common humanity matters more."

—**Bill Clinton**

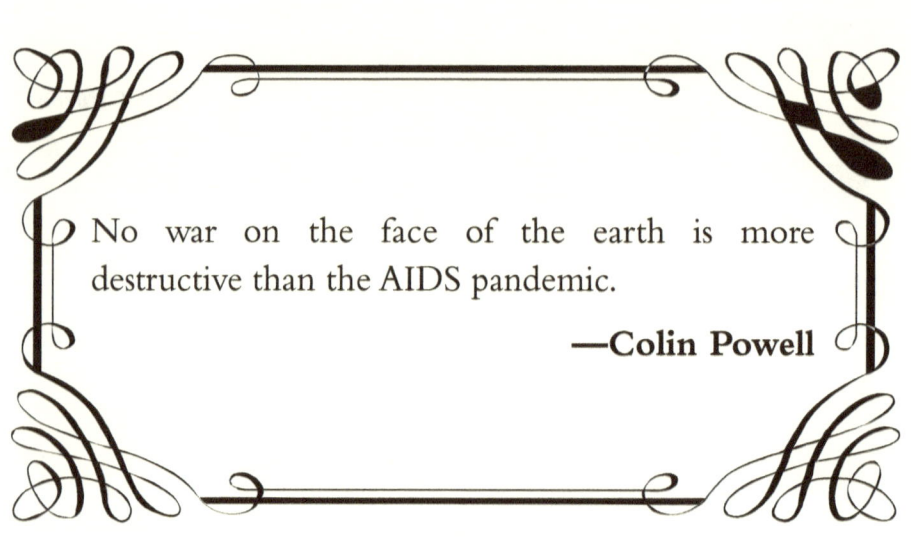

No war on the face of the earth is more destructive than the AIDS pandemic.

—Colin Powell

THE FIGURES

> ➢ Close to 15 million children have lost one or both parents to HIV/AIDS (UNICEF).

> ➢ 230,000 children under the age of 15 died of HIV/AIDS related illnesses in 2011 (amfAR).

> ➢ Between 2009 and 2011 antiretroviral drugs prevented 409,000 children from HIV infection (UNAIDS).

> ➢ There were 2.5 million new cases of HIV in 2011 (CDC).

> ➢ In 2011, 1.1 million people died of HIV/AIDS related causes, bringing the total number of deaths since the pandemic began to 30 million (UNAIDS).

> ➢ Every 9.5 minutes, someone in the U.S. is infected with HIV (AIDS.gov).

> ➢ As many as 5.9 million people in South Africa are living with HIV (UNAIDS).

> ➢ As many as 3.4 Million people in Nigeria are living with the virus (NACA)

> ➢ Bangladesh's HIV/AIDS rate has increased by almost 25% since 2000 (UNAIDS).

> ➢ In 2011, 83,000 children and adults were newly infected with HIV in Latin America (UNAIDS).

> ➢ Estonia has the highest prevalence of HIV/AIDS in Europe (CIA.GOV).

➢ More than 35 million people now live with HIV/AIDS.3.3 million of them are under the age of 15(UNAIDS)

➢ In 2012, an estimated 2.3 million people were newly infected with HIV.260,000 were under the age of 15. (UNAIDS)

Sub-Saharan Africa

More than two-thirds (70 percent) of all people living with HIV; 25 million live in sub-Saharan Africa—including 88 percent of the world's HIV-positive children. In 2012, an estimated 1.6 million people in the region became newly infected. An estimated 1.2 million adults and children died of AIDS, accounting for 75 percent of the world's AIDS deaths in 2012. (UNAIDS)

Asia and the Pacific

In Asia and the Pacific, nearly 351,000 people became newly infected in 2012, bringing the total number of people living with HIV/AIDS there to nearly 5 million. AIDS claimed an estimated 261,000 lives in the region in 2012.

Caribbean

Approximately 12,000 people became newly infected in the Caribbean in 2012, bringing the total number of people living with HIV/AIDS there to more than 250,000. AIDS claimed an estimated 11,000 lives in 2012. (UNAIDS)

Central and South America

There were an estimated 86,000 new HIV/AIDS infections and 52,000 AIDS-related deaths in Central and South America in 2012. This region currently has 1.5 million people living with HIV/AIDS. (UNAIDS)

North Africa and the Middle East

Approximately 260,000 people are living with HIV in this region and an estimated 32,000 people became newly infected in 2012. An estimated 17,000 adults and children died of AIDS. (UNAIDS)

Eastern Europe and Central Asia

Some 130,000 people were newly infected with HIV in 2012, bringing the number of people living with HIV/AIDS to 1.3 million. HIV/AIDS claimed 91,000 lives in 2012. (UNAIDS)

Western and Central Europe

In 2012, there were 29,000 new cases of HIV, bringing the number of people living with HIV in Western and Central Europe to 860,000. An estimated 7,600 people in these regions died of AIDS in 2012.

Quote

"We all pray not to be the next addition to the AIDS statistics, but we need act sincerely to ensure those prayers are answered"

—**Oche Otorkpa**

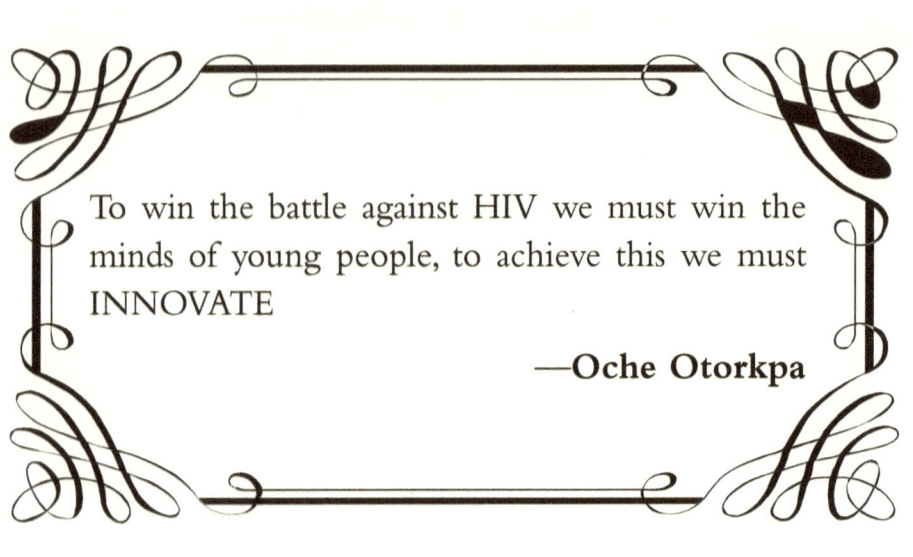

To win the battle against HIV we must win the minds of young people, to achieve this we must INNOVATE

—Oche Otorkpa

EPILOGUE

In the end we must come to the realisation that none of us is immune from the dangers posed by the disease, in an increasingly interdependent world, it is important that we come to terms with the reality that unless we change our approach, rethink our strategies and evolve new and innovative ways of confronting the challenge we will continue to play catch up with the virus.

Let it be said, that the future will continue to look bleak.

Until, corrupt officials stop seeing the Virus as a money spinning machine.

Until, Non Governmental Organizations and civil society groups live up to their responsibilities.

Until, hospital and laboratories across the globe ensure best practices and next practices.

Until, parents and guardians see the need to discuss taboo subjects.

Until, we stop pampering our societies with the aim of achieving behavioural change.

Until, we see the need to sacrifice certain aspects of our lifestyles.

Until, we see the need for care and support for those living with the virus.

Until, we stop chasing shadows and start innovating.

Until, we come to accept the fact that although we might have lost several battles the WAR could still be WON.

"Over to you"

ABOUT THE AUTHOR

Oche Joseph Otorkpa is a Microbiologist, an Integrated Disease Surveillance and Response (IDSR) specialist, and a winner of the UNICEF/NYSC Peer Educators award. He works with Students, Religious organizations, cities and communities engaging young people in the Conceptualization, Design, and Implementation of programmes and activities that seek to enhance the protection of the girl child as well as the promotion of the reproductive health agenda. A regular guest speaker at events. He is happily married to Dr Chinenye Otorkpa a Family physician and they live in Lokoja, Nigeria.

ABOUT THE BOOK

This book, a collection of stories on the lives of HIV carriers was inspired by a taxi driver who once told the author that if he knew one percent of what people infected with HIV go through, he would have done all within his power to avoid being infected.

REVIEWS

Indeed a very well written mini book highlighting the dark side of HIV/AIDS touching crucial aspects of Human greed, value system, drug menace, teenage motherhood, sex trafficking, sex abuse, exploitation of children, the suffering of women and children and the courage of women to fight this evil along with some eye opening statistics.

Let this book become part a movement in terms of guiding teens where sex education is a taboo, reinforcing the right value system and making society more responsible towards women and children.

I am sure this book will compel many to think and change their lives for a better future. By this you are doing a great service to your society, nation and mankind at large.

Vikas P. Chawda

Founder, CEO Quantum Leap India

REFERENCES

Project MK NAOMI, http://en.wikipedia.org/wiki/Project_ MKNAOMI (Accessed 8-11-13)

Statistics on Teen Pregnancy http://www.teenshelter.org/ Jims_Statistics_on_Teenage_Pregnancy_11-11-06.pdf PAGES 1-3 (Accessed 8-11-13)

Reproductive Health and Early Life Changes http://web.unfpa.org/ intercenter/cycle/earlylife.htm (Accessed 8-11-13)

J. virol. (1988) Simian immunodeficiency virus from African green monkeys Journal of Virology. November; 62(11): 4123-4128.

Endocarditis Risk factors, http://www.mayoclinic.com/health/ endocarditis/DS00409/DSECTION=risk-factors (Accessed 8-11-13)

Manual For Peer Educators (2003) Abuja: United Nations Children Fund.

Conference of the Parties to the Convention against Trans-national Organized Crime (2011) Working Group on Trafficking in Persons, CTOC/COP/WG.4/2011/3, Analysis of key concepts: focus on the concept of "abuse of power or of a position of vulnerability" in article 3 of the Protocol to Prevent, Suppress and Punish Trafficking in Persons, Especially Women and Children, supplementing the United Nations Convention against Transnational Organized Crime, Background paper prepared by the Secretariat.

Eastern Europe and Central Asia http://www.unaids.org/en/ regionscountries/regions/easterneuropeandcentralasia/ (Accessed 15-11-13)

Every minute, a young woman is newly infected with HIV http://www.unaids.org/en/resources/infographics/20120608gendereveryminute/(Accessed 15-11-13)

Why Mosquitoes Cannot Transmit AIDS. http://www.rci.rutgers.edu/~insects/aids.htm (Accessed 18-11-13)

Male Latex Condoms and Sexually Transmitted Diseases. http://www.cdc.gov/condomeffectiveness/brief.html (Accessed 18-11-13)

Clark, M.A. (2008) Vulnerability, Prevention and Human Trafficking: The Need for a new Paradigm. In United Nations Office on Drugs and Crime, An Introduction to Human Trafficking: Vulnerability, Impact and Action, Vienna, UNODC.

Global report on Trafficking in persons 2012

http://www.unodc.org/documents/dataananalysis/glotip/Trafficking_in_Persons_2012_web.pdf (Accessed 18-11-13)

Ciconte, E. (2005). The trafficking flows and routes of Eastern Europe, WEST Project ref. N. 2A071. Bologna, WEST.

Estabrooks, G.H. Hypnosis comes of age. Science Digest, 44-50, April 1971

Gillmor, D. I Swear By Apollo. Dr. Ewen Cameron and the CIA-Brainwashing Experiments. Montreal: Eden press, 1987.

Scheflin, A.W., & Opton, E.M. The Mind manipulators. New York: Paddington Press, 1978.

Thomas, G. Journey into Madness. The Secret Story of Secret CIA Mind Control and Medical Abuse. New York: Bantam, 1989 (paperback 1990).

Weinstein, H. Psychiatry and the CIA: Victims of Mind Control. Washington, DC: American Psychiatric Press, 1990.

"Of Dart Guns and Poisons". *Time*. 1975-09-29. Retrieved 2007-01-29.

What HIV/AIDS Can Do to Education, and What Education Can Do to HIV/AIDS. http://sedosmission.org/old/eng/kelly_1.htm (Accessed 18-11-13)

Ainsworth, M. & Semali, I. (1998) Who is Most Likely to Die of AIDS? Socioeconomic Correlates of Adult Deaths in Kagera Region, Tanzania. In Confronting AIDS: Evidence from the Developing World (eds. M. Ainsworth, L. Fransen, & M. Over). Brussels: The European Commission.

Beare, H., Caldwell, B. J. & Millikan, R. H. (1989) Creating an Excellent School. Some New Management Techniques. London: Routledge.

Filmer, D. (1998) The Socioeconomic Correlates of Sexual behaviour: A Summary of Results from an Analysis of DHS Data. In Confronting AIDS: Evidence from the Developing World (eds. M. Ainsworth, L. Fransen, & M. Over). Brussels: The European Commission.

Fylkesnes, K., Musonda, R. M., Sichone, M., Ndhlovu, Z., Tembo, F., Monze, M., Kaetano, L., Malamba, C., Phiri, S., & Mwakamui, C. (1999) "Favourable Changes in the HIV Epidemic in Zambia in the 1990s". Late Breaker Abstract for XI—ICASA, the Eleventh International Conference on AIDS and STDs in Africa, Mulungushi International Conference Centre, Lusaka, 12-16 September, 1999.

Greenfield, T. (1991) Re-forming and Re-valuing Educational Administration. Whence and When Cometh the Phoenix. In T. Greenfield & P. Ribbins (eds.) (1993) Greenfield on Educational Administration. London: Routledge.

MOE (Ministry of Education) (1996) Educating Our Future. National Policy on Education. Lusaka: Ministry of Education.

Oxfam (1999) Education Now. Break the Cycle of Poverty. Oxford: Oxfam International.

Shaeffer, S. (1994) The Impact of HIV/AIDS on Education: A Review of Literature and Experience. Background Paper Presented to an IIEP Seminar, Paris, 8-10 December, 1993. Paris: International Institute for Educational Planning.

Siame, Y. (1998) Youth Alive Zambia. BCP (Behavioural Change Programme) Experience. Ndola: Mission Press.

UNAIDS (1997) Impact of HIV and Sexual Health Education on the Sexual Behaviour of Young People: A Review Update. Geneva: UNAIDS (Joint United Nations Programme on HIV/AIDS).

(1998) HIV/AIDS and Human Rights. International Guidelines. Geneva: UNAIDS.

(1999a) Listen, Learn, Live! World AIDS Campaign with Children and Young People. Facts and Figures. Geneva: UNAIDS.

(1999b) Listen, Learn, Live! World AIDS Campaign with Children and Young People. Key Issues and Ideas for Action. Geneva: UNAIDS.

World Bank (1999) Intensifying Action Against HIV/AIDS in Africa: Responding to a Development Crisis. Africa Region, The World Bank. Washington, DC: The World Bank:

This is serious monkey business. http://seriousmonkeybusiness.wordpress.com/2011/05/17/siv-to-hiv-monkeying-around-with-an-epidemic/(Accessed 18-11-13)

lthaus, C.L. & De Boer, R.J. (2008). Dynamics of Immune Escape during HIV/SIV Infection. PLoS Comput Biol, 4(7).

Blancou, P., Vartanian, J.P., Christopherson, C., Chenciner, N., Basilico, C., Kwok, S., & Wain-Hobson, S. (2001). Polio vaccine samples not linked to AIDS. Science, 410(6832): 1045.

Chitnis, A., Rawls, D., & Moore, J. (2000). Origin of HIV Type 1 in Colonial French Equatorial Africa? AIDS Res & Lentiviruses, 16(1): 5-8.

Gao, F., Yue, L., White, A.T., Pappas, P.G., Barchue, J., Hanson, A.P., Greene, B.M., Sharp, P.M., Shaw, G.M., & Hahn, B.H. (1992). Human infection by genetically diverse SIVsmm-related HIV-2 in West Africa. Nature, 358: 495-499.

Gao, F., Bailes, E., Robertson, D.L., Chen, Y., Rodenburg, C.M., Michael, S.F., Cummins, L.B., Arthur, L.O., Peeters, M., Shaw, G.M., Sharp, P.M., & Hahn, B.H. (1999). Origin of HIV-1 in the chimpanzee, Pan troglodytes troglodytes. Nature, 397: 436-441.

Simian immunodeficiency virus
http://en.wikipedia.org/wiki/Simian_immunodeficiency_virus
(Accessed 18-11-13)

Peeters, M.; Courgnaud, V.; Abela, B. (2001). "Genetic Diversity of Lentiviruses in Non-Human Primates". *AIDS Reviews* **3**: 3-10. Retrieved 2010-09-19.

Peeters, M.; Courgnaud, V. (2002). "Overview of Primate Lentiviruses and their Evolution in Non-human Primates in Africa". In C. Kuiken, B. Foley, E. Freed, B. Hahn, B. Korber, P. A. Marx, F. E. McCutchan, J. W. Mellors, and S. Wolinsky. HIV sequence compendium. Los Alamos, NM: Theoretical Biology and Biophysics Group, Los Alamos National Laboratory. pp. 2-23. Retrieved 2010-09-19

Donald G. McNeil, Jr. (September 16, 2010). "Precursor to H.I.V. Was in Monkeys for Millennia". New York Times. Retrieved 2010-09-17. "In a discovery that sheds new light on the history of AIDS, scientists have found evidence that the ancestor to the virus that causes the disease has been in monkeys and apes for at least 32,000 years—not just a few hundred years, as had been previously thought. . . . That means humans have presumably been exposed many times to S.I.V., the simian immunodeficiency virus, because people have been hunting monkeys for millenniums, risking infection every time they butcher one for food."

Worobey, Michael; Telfer, Paul; Souquière, Sandrine; Hunter, Meredith; Coleman, Clint A.; Metzger, Michael J.; Reed, Patricia; Makuwa, Maria et al. (2010). "Island Biogeography Reveals the Deep History of SIV". *Science* **329** (5998): 1487. Bibcode:2010Sci . . . 329.1487W. doi:10.1126/science.1193550. PMID 20847261.

Kestler, H.; Kodama, T.; Ringler, D.; Marthas, M.; Pedersen, N.; Lackner, A.; Regier, D.; Sehgal, P.; Daniel, M.; King, N.; Et, A. (1990). "Induction of AIDS in rhesus monkeys.

Peer care and support network improves quality of life of women and families affected by HIV in Ruili City, Yunnan Province, China newsletter.childrenandaids.org/peer-care-and-support-network-improves-quality-of-life-of-women-and-families-affected-by-hiv-in-ruili-city-yunnan-province-china (Accessed on 24-11-2013)

Forcible Rape. www.fbi.gov/about-us/cjis/ucr/crime-in-the-u.s/2011/crime-in-the-u.s.-2011/violent-crime/forcible-rape#disablemobile (Accessed on 24-11-2013)

Beyond Barbies and Baby Dolls. www.eatingdisorderhope.com/blog/beyond-barbies-and-baby-dolls (Accessed on 24-11-2013)

Statistics highlight link between injecting drug use and HIV
www.unodc.org/unodc/en/frontpage/2009/June/statistics-
emphasize-link-between-injecting-drug-use-and-hiv.html,
(Accessed on 24-11-2013)

Statistics: Worldwide www.amfar.org/about-hiv-and-aids/
facts-and-stats/statistics—worldwide/(Accessed on 24-11-2013)

www.ingramcontent.com/pod-product-compliance
Lightning Source LLC
Chambersburg PA
CBHW020537290526
45786CB00002B/915